AF740783

Autism Spectrum Disorder

Autism Spectrum Disorder

Perspectives from Psychoanalysis and Neuroscience

Susan P. Sherkow, MD

and

Alexandra M. Harrison, MD

With contributions by
William M. Singletary, MD

JASON ARONSON
Lanham • Boulder • New York • Toronto • Plymouth, UK

Published by Jason Aronson
A wholly owned subsidiary of Rowman & Littlefield
4501 Forbes Boulevard, Suite 200, Lanham, Maryland 20706
www.rowman.com

10 Thornbury Road, Plymouth PL6 7PP, United Kingdom

Copyright © 2014 by Jason Aronson

Sherkow, Susan. "The Dyadic Psychoanalytic Treatment of a Toddler with Autism Spectrum Disorder," *Psychoanalytic Inquiry Volume, 31*(3) (May 2011): 252-275. Reprinted by permission of Taylor & Francis Ltd., www.tandfonline.com.

All rights reserved. No part of this book may be reproduced in any form or by any electronic or mechanical means, including information storage and retrieval systems, without written permission from the publisher, except by a reviewer who may quote passages in a review.

British Library Cataloguing in Publication Information Available

Library of Congress Cataloging-in-Publication Data

Sherkow, Susan P., 1944– author.
Autism spectrum disorder : perspectives from psychoanalysis and neuroscience / Susan P. Sherkow and Alexandra M. Harrison ; with contributions by William Singletary.
p. ; cm.
Includes bibliographical references and index.
ISBN 978-0-7657-0862-5 (cloth : alk. paper)—ISBN 978-0-7657-0863-2 (electronic)
I. Harrison, Alexandra, 1945– author. II. Singletary, William, contributor. III. Title. [DNLM: 1. Child Development Disorders, Pervasive—therapy. 2. Child. 3. Models, Neurological. 4. Psychoanalytic Therapy—methods. WS 350.8.P4]
RJ51.D48
618.92'85882—dc23
2013034081

∞™ The paper used in this publication meets the minimum requirements of American National Standard for Information Sciences Permanence of Paper for Printed Library Materials, ANSI/NISO Z39.48-1992.

Printed in the United States of America

Contents

List of Figures

List of Tables

Preface

William M. Singletary, MD

For many years, psychoanalysis and neurobiology have been in completely opposite camps regarding the understanding and treatment of autism. We psychoanalysts, as well as others in the field, have been in our own private worlds, not interacting or communicating, something we hope to begin to correct with this book. However, recently Autism Spectrum Disorder (ASD) has become a major public health problem that demands multidisciplinary collaboration. Fortunately, over the past several years, there has been a remarkable confluence of findings from many disciplines, which has made possible the construction of an integrative model of ASD as a neurodevelopmental disorder with psychological and behavioral consequences, which are potentially treatable. Most importantly there seems to be a developing consensus among neurobiological researchers in the field of autism that there are many *different* neurobiological problems that interfere with the functioning of the social brain and therefore lead to autism (Amaral, Rubenstein, & Rogers, 2008).

Of crucial significance, Martha Herbert (Herbert, 2005a, 2005b, 2010; Anderson, Hooker, & Herbert, 2008; Herbert & Anderson, 2008; Herbert & Weintraub, 2012) has developed a new multi-system biological model of autism with emphasis on dynamic, ongoing, reversible impairments of multiple aspects of brain function instead of fixed, genetic, brain defects resulting in irremediable behavioral disturbances. In Herbert's (Herbert & Weintraub, 2012) model, pathophysiology operates at a number of biological (e.g., neuroinflammation and immune function) as well as psychological (e.g., stress) levels and across time, raising the possibility for therapeutic intervention at many points. The recognition that significant improvements in function, including loss of diagnosis, may occur in some children with autism raises realistic hope for recovery (Helt et al., 2008; Dawson, 2008). Geraldine Dawson's (2008) model is another pivotal development. Dawson posits that neurobiological, for example, genetic, *risk factors* contribute to maladaptive patterns of relating between child and parents. She considers these ongoing growth-disturbing modes of parent-child interaction to be, in turn, central *risk processes* for the development of the full autism syndrome. Therefore, Dawson considers optimizing parent-child interactions to play a major role in successful early intervention and, with early diagnosis and treatment, perhaps even prevention.

These groundbreaking neurobiological formulations make possible an interdisciplinary dialogue which includes psychoanalysis. While neurobiology informs us about the workings of the brain, psychoanalysis can open a window to the inner world of the ASD child. Understanding the dynamic interplay among biological and psychological processes in autism is of utmost importance. We hope that this volume will help lead to the development of vital interdisciplinary collaboration in ASD research and treatment. Joining forces can make an invaluable contribution to the realization of our shared ultimate goal, optimizing the development and sense of well-being of each child with ASD. In this way, we can all contribute to enabling ASD children and their families to have as happy and as fulfilling lives as possible.

Acknowledgments

I would like to express my gratitude to Rachel Gorman for her generous and scholarly contributions to this project, to Susannah Levin and Kevin Kautzman for their energetic assistance, and to Barbara Rocah and Richard Lipkin for their wise counsel. I am indebted to my loving family for their unwavering support and patience, and to my patients and their families for their courage and inspiration.

Susan P. Sherkow

I am grateful to my husband, David, for his love and support, to my mentors and teachers Anni Bergman, Ed Tronick, and Gilbert Kliman, and to the teachers at the Cambridge Ellis School. I also wish to express gratitude to the children who have taught me more than I could learn from any book or training, and to their parents, who have allowed me to work with their precious children and to care about them.

Alexandra M. Harrison

I feel deep gratitude to my parents for their love, guidance, and generosity, to my son for his steadfast presence and support in times of need, and to my wife without whom none of this would have been possible. Amy and Tom Smith have been invaluable with their patient technical assistance in editing and with diagrams.

William M. Singletary

The authors join in thanking Anni Bergman, whose groundbreaking work with ASD children has been and continues to be an inspiration. We are particularly grateful for her wisdom, encouragement, and support.

Introduction

OVERVIEW

As psychoanalysts, we feel it is important to bring our experience working with young children diagnosed with Autism Spectrum Disorder (ASD) to parents, clinicians, and educators. Our goal is to offer a guidebook to understanding and treating the ASD child from the dual perspectives of psyche and neurofunction through detailed descriptions of our intensive treatments of four children who began therapy between the ages of two to three. We will explore the possible mechanisms of change at work in their psychoanalytically informed treatments at home, in the office, and in the classroom. We will share the insights we have gained into what it is like to be a child with ASD and what it means to be the parent of such a child.

We use the term "ASD" to refer to those children who present with the classical triad of symptoms: language impairment, social impairment, and repetitive and stereotypic behaviors. We use the term in the most inclusive sense of the diagnosis, because our focus is on the primary neurobiological and developmental processes that engender the symptoms. In keeping with the broader perspective of assessing and treating this population, we include in our discussions children who do not meet the formal criteria for the diagnosis of ASD but whose behaviors and symptoms display a level of uneven development sufficient to warrant consideration. We will frequently return to this phrase "uneven development" to describe those children who show significant lags or gaps between the acquisitions of competencies. For example, an unevenly developing child might be incredibly verbally precocious but lack social awareness or computational skills to a debilitating degree.

Psychoanalysis has often been discounted as a treatment for autism and recently has been displaced by therapies that seem more practical, pragmatic, behavioral, and teachable to parents, educators, and therapists. Until now, psychoanalysis for the most part has been disconnected from brain research and the efficacy of behaviorally based therapies. We hope to bridge that disconnection by presenting cases where our psychoanalytic perspective and corresponding techniques were used to treat children with a neurobiological disorder.

With the challenge of treating children with neurobiological disorders in sharp focus, this volume explores the interacting domains of mind, body, and relationships. Just as psychopharmacological drugs change neuronal synapses and alter a patient's mood, we hypothesize that psychoanalysis as a treatment also modifies the biochemistry of the brain, resulting in alteration of emotion and cognition. Our chapter on neurobiological mechanisms of change describes these hypotheses in depth.

We postulate that the symptoms of ASD are behavioral representations of atypically developing neuronal processes. The ASD child, whose neurophysiologic deficits seemed to have interfered with developing an organization of useful symbols and affects to manage actions as well as relationships, behaves as though he lacks understanding of his own mental states and those of others. His inability to integrate experiences and to express himself makes it difficult for his parents to understand him, and vice versa. In addition, the ego seems to compensate by acquiring a repertoire of defense mechanisms inconsistent with flexible adaptations, exacerbating the problem.

We begin by taking the reader through the applicable basic concepts of development: what it must be like for a baby whose wiring has the potential to interfere with his development right from the start. In each section below, we describe the neurotypical picture followed by what we see in our patients and our hypotheses about the intrapsychic, the neurofunctional, and the interpersonal mechanisms of action, and how they relate to one another.

THE DOMAINS OF MIND, BODY, AND RELATIONSHIPS

Psychoanalysis, having been conceived as a theory and treatment of the mind based on biological processes, allows for the perspective of seeing any child in relation to his own unique biological nature while taking into account universal social, motoric, and cognitive expectancies and the acquisition of a hierarchy of skills and competencies. Our work in emphasizing developmental processes continues to be based on the inextricability of mind and body, equally so for a neurotypical child and an ASD child. That the polarized features of "nature" and "nurture" are now thought to be inseparable perspectives of the same process is especially relevant in ASD, where, in our experience, the "uniqueness" of each child is more apparent than the "sameness," despite the triad of diagnostic criteria.

Our developmental perspective focuses also on the way babies grow and learn to become independent and process social information. Winnicott (1958) proposed that a baby learns "who he is" through the gradual development of his experiential state being mirrored in his mother's expression. The processes of internalizing mother's caretaking, in all of its complexity, is governed by interpersonal, reciprocal mechanisms through the creation of mental representations of self and the mother (Jacobson, 1954).

In addition to a child's endowment, the ongoing internalization of mother's actions, emotions, sensations, and attitudes during the critical first three years of life is processed by the sensory, proto-cognitive, and body-bound capacities of each infant. How the infant "reads" his mother and integrates his perceptions of her is most relevant to our understanding the deficits in ASD. Likewise, the ability of a mother to respond to her baby is all-important. "There is no baby without a mother" (Winnicott, 1956). Winnicott (1962) also notably pointed to the impact on the developing toddler of the "good-enough" quality of these interactions, while Fonagy et al. elaborated on the importance of the input by mother, and integration by baby, of being *just* good enough, and not perfect (Fonagy, Gergely, Jurist, & Target, 2002).

Toddler and mother navigate in relative, hopefully "good-enough" synchrony, through the stages of development associated with the acquisition of competence in feeding, toilet training, sleeping, learning, and forming relationships within the family structure. Critical to this process, from birth, is the child's implicit formation of representations of his mother, himself, and his mother-self pair in action. These representations are the bedrock of the child's ability to use symbols to represent his experiences, feelings, and wishes. Symbols appear first in the form of babbling, then words, and then sentences, enabling a child to express his needs, use his budding "imagination" to control his impulses, accept discipline, and feel safe in being understood by his parents. Once having established the ability to use language, a child continues to symbolically process his experiences and his emotional, cognitive, and bodily reactions through elaborated fantasies and pretend play, furthering his sense of mastery of himself and his relationships.

UNDERSTANDING THE ASD CHILD

Applying our psychoanalytic study of development is crucial to understanding ASD toddlers whose learning style may interfere with the essential internalization of mother's ministrations and prevent him from extrapolating from one experience to another, thus precluding the use of maternal structuring to learn and predict (Qian & Lipkin, 2011). Rather than learning from interpolating from one situation to the next, which allows an infant to scaffold and categorize information, Qian and Lipkin propose that an ASD child acquires disconnected, non-integrated information which is of diminished usefulness in comprehending input from himself or his mother (Qian & Lipkin, 2011). It is likely the child's atypical neurobiology also interferes with his awareness of who mother and father are as functioning people and parents and what they expect (Sherkow, 2005, 2011; Singletary, 2010).

The ASD child's neurobiological differences make it difficult for him to process information (Helt, Kelley, Kinsbourne, Pandey, Boorstein, Herbert, & Fein, 2008). Our case material shows clinical examples of just this kind of interference brought about by a toddler's inability to process *his sense of his mother*, which may be very different from how his mother understands herself, much less how others understand her. From an object-relations perspective, one could describe ASD children as unable to internalize their parents as fully developed objects, as if they were unable to process stimuli at a synaptic level (Helt et al., 2008). Our patients have shown us how ASD toddlers typically appear to be fending off stimulation as though they were being assaulted by internal and external sensory overload, withdrawing into perseverative, robotic, or avoidant activity.

Importantly, one kind of sensory overload we have seen in an ASD child stems from his awareness of his parents' increasing disappointment in him as he fails to meet their expectations. He, in turn, processes his own disappointment in his parents, who are unable to provide him with the sense of being understood and cared for (Sherkow, 2005, 2011). We hypothesize, based on our experience, that our patients seem biologically driven to make "something" happen that they are able to control and so become stuck on actions that seem arbitrary to their parents such as twirling a toy car, using repetitive sounds, or being fixated, as in one of our cases, on something concrete and accessible such as a compact disc. Our impression is that parents' behaviors can seem just as arbitrary to the child.

We have observed that the atypical neuronal processes seem to appear in a child at about 12 to 18 months, just when his parents expect him to be able to use language to express his wishes, needs, and feeling in a social context. Because 12 to 18 months is a critical period in beginning the separation-individuation process, these toddlers may become more than typically clingy and demanding, or, as we will describe, start to become aversive and avoidant. Functionally, the ASD toddler appears to be physiologically unable to process the emerging relationship, behaving as if he is fending off the signals of interpersonal interaction. Moreover, many of the children we have seen appear to be hypersensitive to sounds, sights, smells, or tactile sensations, which further complicates their ability to integrate relational input, and increases the parent's frustration. Not only may these children overreact to sensory stimuli, but they appear to be unable to differentiate between those stimuli that are benign and those that are noxious, often perceiving their parent's behavior, including their attempts to love and soothe, as disruptive, rather than contributing to the child's comfort (Sherkow, 2005, 2011). Mother's ensuing confusion understandably may impair her ability to comprehend her toddler's needs in both the domains of self-expression and gratification and in the domain of evolving separation-individuation. As we will show, in the ensuing cycling of mutual frustration, the likelihood of confrontations increases, adding, moreover, to the picture of "terrible 2's," resulting in the toddler's aggressive storms, severe temper tantrums, and/or regression to frightening bouts of biting, head-banging, or hair-pulling.

Whether our patients were ASD or had uneven development, we have seen that the ability of the toddler to develop self-regulation, and to trust and make use of his parent to aid in developmental tasks, has been markedly interrupted. Helt et al. (2008) refer to a neurobiological "core limitation" in these children, which prevents them from experiencing social and language input from their environment, and interferes with primary motivation, a basic function that drives neurotypical children to attend to environmental stimulation and learning. Helt et al. (2008) point to a "sticky" or hyperfocused attention that leads these children to being avoidant or "stuck."

Accordingly, it is often very difficult for this parent population to know how to set appropriate expectations for, and to discipline, our young patients. Often parents will either expect their child to comply with demands beyond his capacities, or they will take over tasks their child is now ready to handle himself.

THEORY OF MIND AND THE MAKING OF MEANING

The brain constantly processes meaning. Mental activity, every thought, action, dream, and conversation, is not only processed in the "real world" but is also processed through invisible activity of the brain. Indeed, the key word here is "processing," essential to understanding how children make meaning of their implicit and explicit experiences. The developmental researchers Tronick and Harrison (2007) propose that patterns of internal development emerge simultaneously in multiple domains, both implicit and explicit. A child's experiences of past and present interactions combine to promote relatively predictable readings of the world and of one's self, as well as differentiate between what is "known" and "unknown," and allow novel experiences to be integrated.

How patterns fail to materialize is speculative, addressed in many areas of research. One possibility is that, following Fonagy et al. (2002), the problem lies in an infant's "reading" his mother's intentions and affects; the other, following Qian and Lipkin's learning theories, is that the problem lies in his categorizing what he "reads" (Fonagy, 2002; Qian & Lipkin 2011). For example, can we understand at the neuronal level how a baby makes predictable meaning of his mother's appearance with a bottle, and thus will stop crying when she walks in the door, "reading" her arrival as an accurate representation of reality? Would his failure to do so arise from a deficit, namely being unable to categorize a pattern from her previous arrivals and thus no comforting could ensue? In other words, he is not integrating his "like" experiences. Or, alternatively, is he unable to read her arrival as potentially comforting, and therefore unable to make meaning of her behavior, seeing each arrival as novel? In either case, the neurofunctional outcome is an inability to make meaningful assessments and integrations of those representations.

The meaning-making processes in ASD appear to be impaired by atypical neuronal wiring. How babies neurobiologically represent and make meaning of their experience is not known. Neither do we know how atypical wiring affects the meaning-making processes in ASD (Fonagy & Target, 1998; Fonagy et al., 2002). Fonagy proposes that making meaning begins through an innate capacity to "mentalize," which is the ability to form mental representations of one's own feelings, experiences, thoughts, and intentions, as well as imaging what one understands about another person's state of mind, feelings, and experiences (Fonagy et al., 2002).

Additionally, work in the area of Theory of Mind proposes that a child must have a theory of another person's mind as a precondition for making meaning of one's own or another's mind, implying that there is an unconscious mechanism that allows a child to distinguish between himself and another (Klin & Jones, 2007). Baron-Cohen (1995) applies this framework for the development of meaning-making. His "Theory of Shared Attention Mechanism" (SAM) maintains that "you and an agent see and experience the same thing"—in effect, a pointing mechanism (Baron-Cohen, 1995, p. 46). Emphasizing that biologically, "the chief aspect of SAM is to create a 'drive' to share, to get on someone's wavelength," he builds a model of understanding the functional impairment in ASD, whereby ASD infants cannot learn to share attention (Baron-Cohen, Leslie, & Firth, 1985). Describing the functional impairment in ASD in his terms, deficits in ASD in this area can lead to the range of social, communicative, and imaginative defects we see in our patients; by interfering with being aware of one's volitional, perceptual, and cognitive mechanisms, our patients have difficulty thinking, knowing, pretending, believing, imagining, dreaming, guessing, and deceiving, all of which are essential to forming a coherent understanding of one's own and others' mental states (Baron-Cohen, 1995).

Putting these two perspectives together, in practice we see in the manifest behavior of a child who is developing unevenly, or has ASD, profound deficits that seem to interfere with his development of "Theory of Mind," or schemas, negatively affecting his ability to "mentalize" his mother. In place of creating an imaginative representational world, which would lead to being able to play and pretend (Tustin, 1988; Baron-Cohen, 1995), ASD toddlers seem to be missing the building blocks that would lead to reciprocal understanding between mother and child of each other's feelings and thoughts, and thus create a platform for building basic trust. Instead, ASD children are observed to be unable to understand their own minds or the minds of their mothers, and become increasingly preoccupied with perseverative, concrete activity that serves the opposite goal, to fend off relating as if it were a form of aversive stimulation, by retreating into avoidant mannerisms. For many children, it would seem that their withdrawal from mother comes about because their mothers' fear of their symptomatic behavior is yet one more form of overstimulation (Sherkow, 2011; Dawson, 2008). Importantly, the functions of mentalizing and sharing joint attention rest on being individuated to the extent that one sees the "other" as a separate person, and mutually having the ability to impact upon another's thoughts and feelings. This is a crucial step in the direction of acquiring empathy, and an essential ingredient in developing the capacity for forming symbols, language, impulse control, and imaginary and pretend play (Fonagy & Target, 1998; Baron-Cohen, 1995).

The children we describe herein exemplify the inability to mentalize (read and categorize) their mother's intentions. From the neurofunctional point of view, we could hypothesize that such an inability in turn interferes with their ability to extrapolate from one experience to the next, thus not building an ability to anticipate or navigate transitions, whether benign or threatening. This inevitably makes it hard for them to make predictions from their everyday experience, a competency necessary for self-regulation and hence independence, and for acquiring a repertoire of coping mechanisms consistent with flexible adaptations. Our cases will also illustrate how these children are unable to master states of overarousal brought about by their inability to use anticipatory anxiety to manage transitions, an extension of their overall inability to apply cognitive mechanisms, categorical learning, and interpolated learning for the purpose of integrating internal and external messages (Qian & Lipkin, 2011). The inability to discriminate mother's behaviors, commands, wishes, and moods appears to evoke a need for a concrete and predictable substitute for the soothing qualities of mothering. We conjecture that a secondary gain for the choice of a concrete object is that it is impervious to the child's frustration, fear, and aggression.

WHY PSYCHOANALYSIS? FANTASY AND THE UNCONSCIOUS

Psychoanalytic training teaches students how to understand conscious behavior, thoughts, ideas, social relationships, and the unconscious and defensive mechanisms that *motivate* human behavior. Psychoanalysts base their knowledge on intensive study of the developmental trajectory from infancy through adulthood and old age. We examine the complexity of interpersonal interactions and explore intrapersonal conflicts in which one may be struggling with frightening or unacceptable aspects of oneself.

We assume the integrative process offered by psychoanalytically informed treatment optimizes the capacity for the therapist to address, explore, and repair the apparent missing neuronal connections that we hypothesize affect self-regulation, cognition, and object relations (Herbert & Weintraub, 2012; Dawson, 2008). Our psychoanalytic perspective compels us to be particularly attuned to how missing neuronal connections may impact the integration of aggressive forces in early brain development, with respect to both "agency" and impulses, and how that integration manifests itself in the psychological organization of an ASD child. Aggressive feelings, after all, and their derivatives are amongst the most basic emotions in the developing infant. How an ASD child expresses and manages his assertive and aggressive impulses is integral to our understanding of the psychodynamics of each child, as well as to our understanding the experience of each evolving mother/child relationship and their mutual relationship within their social sphere.

Functionally, the basic aim of every therapy for a child with ASD or uneven development is to ameliorate his symptoms, whether through addressing his needs for developing language skills, social skills, or reduction in or elimination of idiosyncratic behaviors. In addition to focusing on helping a child change his behaviors and acquire missing competencies, many therapeutic modalities also endeavor to improve a child's relationship to his family and society by helping him and his parents *understand* his behavior, motivations, and feelings.

An analytically trained interactive partner, whether a parent, caregiver, educator, or other specialist who works with ASD children can aim much deeper, informed by a psychoanalytic, developmental perspective. Analytically trained specialists add to their repertoire attention to the unconscious. The unconscious is at work in the formation of conflicts and fantasies, which influence behavior, including ASD behavior. An ASD child is just as likely to worry about preferring one parent over another, or experience sibling rivalry, as a neurotypical child. The difference is that most treatments do not address the exquisitely detailed process by which a child develops his thoughts and ideas or how the unconscious wishes, fears, and fantasies influence his thinking and behavior and impact his ability to form and maintain relationships.

Indeed, the increasing number of identified cases of ASD in the past ten years has led to a new parental, educational, and public awareness of the needs of an expanding population of pre-teens and teenagers who are socially at risk. These teenagers feel ill-equipped to leave the safety net of their parents and move into "group" relationships and often know neither how to navigate the typical issues of puberty, competitiveness, and formation of ego ideals nor how to set appropriate education and career goals (Sherkow, 2013). Development does not end in childhood or adolescence. A psychoanalytic perspective can be used at every developmental age to assist the ASD population in navigating self-regulatory challenges from the demands of society.

THE PSYCHOANALYTIC MODEL OF PLAY

As psychoanalysts, we are not daunted by behaviors in our patients that may appear to be "nonsense," meaningless, threatening, or mysterious. Each of us has found our own techniques to search for meaning, patterns, and/or conflicts embedded in a child's presentation. Whether examining play, language, or parent-child interactions, we will show how the psychoanalyst explores a child's interactions with his environment: how, why, and under what conditions he processes information, and how these processes interconnect with cognition and emotion for both the child and his parents. Because a brain is constantly in flux, and given the recent work on neuroplasticity, we can be assured that a psychoanalytic play session has an impact on the brain (Herbert & Weintraub, 2012).

Psychoanalysis involves developing an intimate, dependent relationship with the patient, with the focus on the patient's inner world and the patient-analyst interaction. This allows for deep understanding, both symbolically and in the implicit and nonverbal realm, of the patient's actions and words. This "implicit relational knowing," present in every intensive relationship, is made possible by the analyst's training, the frequency of meetings, and the duration of treatment and has been claimed to be the "something more" than interpretation in therapeutic action (Stern, 1985). This domain of "knowing" is particularly relevant to working with toddlers who cannot yet, or have lost the ability to, express themselves.

With its special attention to personal meaning, the psychoanalytic way of thinking equips a practitioner to help her patients understand and express their internal experience in more complex and flexible ways. This is essential, we feel, for work with children and teenagers on the spectrum, who come to treatment with limited or almost no access to their inner world of ideas, feelings, and representations of experience. As we will show in our clinical cases, we focus on helping our patients develop a Theory of Mind and the richness offered by the world of complex perceptions, imagination and a fantasy life, and engagement with family and the outside world.

We will describe dyadic work, which in our vernacular means sitting on the floor in a playroom with a mother and her toddler, surrounded by options for play, but focusing intensively on the engagement between all three partners. We will narrate our work in depth, explaining as we go how the interactions of toddler, parent, and analyst work toward making meaning and creating integration of emotions and thoughts through action, an essential ingredient in learning (Barry, 2000). In the cases we will present, either the parent is in the room during the play sessions and has the opportunity to hear and watch the analyst interact with her child, or there is frequent exchange of information with parents and teachers, as well as interaction with peers.

Often a parent must also translate for her child, whose language is primitive, diminished, or lacking altogether, and whose speech is difficult for a stranger to understand. The analyst may try to narrate the meaning she makes of the child's play, simultaneously enhancing the parent's understanding of the child's mind. At the same time, the analyst assesses the responses both of the child and of the parent, using her own emerging understanding of the child's meanings. In this relational context the child is helped to develop a communication system that uses symbols—both in the direct use of language and in the "language of play"—while simultaneously supporting the growth of empathic relationships with significant others (Bergman, 2004). Indeed, the elaboration of increasingly complex play promotes the experience of a fantasy life that can be appreciated and articulated during the course of the narrative and play work.

A MULTI-SYSTEM APPROACH TO TREATMENT

We look at every individual with ASD or uneven development as a unique person, each of whom has his own subjective perception of himself and the world around him. We work to help these individuals in their struggle to make coherent sense of their perceptions of the environment, particularly their familial and social environment, and to make meaning out of the world around them, as well as making meaning of thoughts and feelings coming from inside their own minds and bodies. In this meaning-making process, we are in effect building new competencies in the vital areas of familial and social function.

Our approach to ASD and uneven development is to think of them as multi-system disorders, to which the application of a multi-system psychobiological model offers the best alternative for a good outcome. Using this treatment model, we can achieve the best possible understanding of the nature of the respective disorder and then choose from an array of modalities with which to treat the child's potentially reversible impairments. Again, we think in terms of an integrative approach for any given child across all treatment paradigms.

We have seen excellent results from integrating psychoanalytic therapy into the other treatments an ASD child receives, to create a coherent and innovative paradigm. Indeed, from our experience, as well as that of other clinicians—including those not involved in psychoanalytic work—we recommend that children on the spectrum need a minimum of 25 hours per week of consistent therapeutic input. This would include dyadic home-based intervention that models and reinforces the dynamic therapy, and OT/PT and speech therapy as needed.

As we will illustrate with our cases, the addition of a psychoanalytically based therapy to an overall treatment protocol adds a particular dimension to the treatment. This dimension is comprised of a profound understanding of the child's internal world—his unconscious mind as well as his conscious functioning—an understanding of his family relationships, and an understanding of the intertwining threads of his development and the roles his parents have played in his growth. Because of this contribution and because of the central integrative function of the analyst in psychodynamic work, the psychoanalyst is well positioned to take on the challenging task of integrating the multiple services a child receives along with psychoanalytic interventions with a *focus on the unique internal experience of the individual person.*

THE EXPERIENCE OF HAVING AN ASD CHILD

There are comparable similarities and differences among the families of children with ASD, parallel to those among the children themselves. In our experience, having a child who does not respond warmly and reciprocally to expressions of interest and love on the part of the parents creates a sense of profound loss and humiliation (Sherkow, 2011). In fact, the rate of depression in the mothers of ASD children is disproportionately high (Carter, Mayes, & Pajer, 1990). Often brothers and sisters of these children resent the enormous investment of parental time and energy required to care for the sibling with ASD. Also, families have different resources with which to face these challenges: some families can afford expensive therapeutic interventions and nannies to take the child to appointments whereas other families must rely on fewer and less expensive interventions and must take the child to the appointments themselves, interrupting their work week and traveling long distances. Thus, the meaning of being the parent or the sibling of a child with ASD varies greatly from family to family.

We believe that the parent-child relationship should be a central focus of all therapeutic interventions for children with ASD and uneven development. In addition, insights from knowledge of childhood experiences of the parent can be brought to bear on the understanding of current family relationship patterns (Freud, 1962). A child analyst treats the entire family system and not the child alone, even if the treatment is an individual analysis plus parent work.

One compelling example is the analyst's potential for helping to manage the family's resources, on all levels, as part of the intervention. It is difficult for all parents of ASD children, desperate for help, to negotiate the marketplace of therapies claiming to offer effective treatment of ASD—multiple types of behavior therapies, special diets, medications, and so forth.

Studies in biological fields have captured the imagination of the general public to a remarkable degree. Parents of children with ASD often become confused by the disparate and sometimes contradictory approaches advertised. These can be so persuasive that parents often feel caught between devoting an unreasonable amount of family resources to the care of their ASD child and feeling anxious or guilty about missing a critical therapeutic opportunity. A child analyst must be prepared to approach all suggested alternative interventions with an open mind, and indeed keep as up to date as possible on developing research, in order to assist the parents with making hard choices about therapy for their child, while also attending to the "family economy"—meaning the time and money devoted to this one child.

FINAL COMMON PATHWAY

It is our point of view that autistic symptoms, regardless of etiology, represent a final common pathway of processes that fail to establish adequate communication and empathy between child and caregivers. This connection is difficult to repair or grow. Typically, the autistic child has moved onto an atypical developmental trajectory, having at some point lost the ability to communicate his needs and feelings to his parents. In turn, the parents have understandably reacted with fear, anxiety, disappointment, frustration, and remorse (Sherkow, 2005, 2011).

Over time, the analytic work increasingly includes the creation of meaningful connections that make sense of the child's experience in the parent-child relationships, and the child's relationships with important others in his world. Given the intensity of a treatment which also includes parents, the analyst can support the parents as a team leader in assessing the efficacy of other concurrent therapies, integrating those therapies, directing parents to additional resources, and helping them to set priorities in the allocation of family resources in treatment planning.

It is important to note that working from a psychoanalytic perspective does not involve trying to "cure" individuals with ASD. Instead, a psychoanalytic treatment aims to build developmental competencies, and to help individuals restore themselves to a healthier developmental path, ultimately creating a life that includes adequate regulation of attention, affects, and motor activity; competency in representing their inner world in symbolic forms, especially language, and the capacity for reciprocal relationships.

ORGANIZATION OF THE BOOK

Our book is divided into several parts, each offering a unique contribution. We introduce our work with a section on dyadic treatment. We will describe our goals in dyadic treatment, and present the analytically informed treatments of Johnny, a child who came to treatment at age 30 months; Corey, who came to treatment at age 25 months; Ethan, who began treatment at 26 months; and Dahlia, who began treatment at age 3 years. The three boys were seen four times per week in the presence of their mothers. They are distinguished in that Johnny was diagnosed as autistic, and lost the diagnosis by age 4. Corey was also diagnosed as autistic, and achieved somewhat fewer mainstream competencies. Ethan was observed to demonstrate "uneven development" with some features that had led him to be misdiagnosed as autistic at age 24 months, with significant consequences. Our next section describes the treatment of Dahlia, age 3, in which both dyadic therapy in the analyst's office and Reflective Network Therapy, a school-based analytic treatment, were combined (Kliman, 2011).

The next section introduces a review of the literature examining the neurobiological perspectives on ASD. It includes sections on the paths to ASD, genetic and epigenetic mechanisms, environmental factors, neuroanatomical factors, neuromodulators and neurotransmitters, neural networks, and neuroplasticity. Finally, we will provide a discussion and integration of our work. At the end, we will consider some of the questions yet to be answered.

CONCLUSION

Not only is this book an attempt to address the complexity of autistic spectrum disorder and uneven development, but it also aims to convey the complexity of the individuals who suffer from the disabilities or disadvantages associated with these clinical entities, a daunting task. As psychoanalysts, we are accustomed to managing complexity and are sometimes frustrated when we encounter reductive formulations for autism and its treatment, or promises, explicit or implicit, of easy cures. Although new and important information about autism in the biological sciences is now available for all to learn and understand, and the technical skills of psychoanalysis—in play and talk therapy—are at our disposal, the integration of the two domains is still a great challenge. Unless we choose a reductive path comparable to that which frustrates us in other related clinical fields, we must shoulder the burden of this integration (Dawson, 2008).

I

Dyadic Therapy

Chapter One

Introduction to Dyadic Work with Toddlers

In this section we will present three case studies of intensive treatment in which we worked with a toddler and mother in dyadic therapy, specifically applying the general model to the population of ASD toddlers brought to us between the ages of 25 to 30 months. In our model, the analyst interacts simultaneously with an infant and his parent in a playroom setting; in the cases we describe, most of the sessions took place with the toddler's mother, although occasionally father or both parents were in attendance. Generally the sessions took place on the floor of a playroom, where the mother and analyst sat on the floor, in the midst of toys, allowing the toddler to set his own agenda. In our method, there are no demands made upon the child or mother nor protocol instructions of any kind. The analyst is an active participant in both play and conversation with toddler and mother, observing, listening, and interacting at all times during an approximately hour-long session. The analyst's objective in dyadic therapy is to observe *while participating*, to formulate meanings based on observations, contribute interventions based on these formulations, and then to observe the associations in play and conversation that follow from the intervention. Indeed, the analyst watches and listens for "play associations" in the same manner one listens for an adult's associations to an analytic interpretation on the couch.

From the outset of the evaluation of a toddler and his family, the analyst assesses each ASD child by applying her knowledge of developmental trajectories and her analytic understanding of the expectable dynamics between infant and parent. Given that each ASD child is unique and neurobiologically complex, we appraise each child's distinct blend of competencies, delays, and symptoms, as well as his family's structure and their strengths and weaknesses. Precisely because the toddler's brain *and* his family network will continue to develop in ways we cannot predict, even as we work together, we believe that our use of dyadic therapy offers a most important advantage in a treatment plan.

Working in dyadic therapy is similar in another way to working with an adult analysand and is an extension of working with children in analysis, in that the analyst's mind ideally hovers over the activity on the floor in a free-floating mode. In addition, having ideally 4-times-per-week exposure to the toddler and his mother, the analyst has access in minute detail to the child's behaviors, the mother/child interactions, and their enactments reflected in their interactions with the therapist. This affords the analyst access to making meaning in every respect, our all-important avenue to useable interventions.

Importantly, in her hovering sensitivity to the myriad intertwining interactions between analyst, toddler, and mother, the analyst can safely help both mother and child with the inevitable frustrations, conflicts, and disappointments. Every degree of angry, stubborn, and hostile feelings inevitably become enacted in the office. The analyst enables the toddler to find meaning in his symptoms, whether in his aversive behavior, repetitive actions or sounds, or outbursts of emotion, while also being able to impart the possible meanings of his behaviors to his mother. The three partners in effect co-create meaning by sharing each other's observations and reactions, translating and adding to the toddler's growing repertoire of meaningful actions and communication.

In effect, the analyst is also free to offer support, guidance, structure, and education as well as playing the opposite role. When appropriate, she can also remain passive, in a reflective role, allowing disorganization and messing, exploration of bodily interest and derivatives of hostile rage, regression along developmental lines, and acting out by the mother toward both her child and the analyst. The analyst also plays an important role in building ego and superego in a toddler who may have yet to internalize guilt and shame, and who has few useful defenses in the face of conflict. Making no demands on the child or the parent, the analyst gives both partners the freedom to express their most primitive, narcissistic, and painful emotions without fear of judgment or the requirement to perform, follow any rules, or to be held to any standard of achievement.

Our experience, as described in the introduction to this volume, has shown us that the neurobiological "differences" in brain development have impacted an ASD or unevenly developing child's ability to respond to the social and emotional demands of family life. His parent often comes to us confused and frustrated in trying to understand her child, who has developed behaviors that seem mysterious, irrational, or alarming. In our dyadic work, and in parent meetings outside of the playroom, our goal is not only to address the symptoms in the toddler, but also to help his parents understand their child's intentions, feelings, and defensive withdrawal and thus work with us to promote the development of cognition, object relations, separation-individuation, and self-regulation.

A very significant aspect of therapeutic success comes about by using the mother directly as the agent and recipient of emotions expressed through play, and very importantly she serves as a translator for those toddlers with little or indecipherable speech. Mother can also act as narrator and historian, noticing that as her child develops play sequences, the toddler enacts his experiences from outside the office. Theoretically Mother can begin to hope for change in her child, by both participating in, and watching interactions between the therapist, toddler, and herself. She can take behavioral modeling cues from the therapist, and also regain her footing in trusting in her own parenting, and knowing how her child thinks and feels. It is our experience that the mother and father's inevitable frustrations, anxiety, and aggression importantly impact the ASD child's world such that it often overtaxes the child's ability to cope. It is important to help parents and other family members deal with these affects to avoid secondary complications in the child.

While this volume makes it abundantly clear that Autism Spectrum Disorders and uneven development arise from a neurobiological etiology, nonetheless a mother not only typically feels emotionally responsible for her child's welfare and treatment, but only too often is caught up in his diagnosis in ways that can both help and hurt. Thus, another crucial aspect to working with a dyad is our access to a mother's understandable and unique emotional responses to the diagnosis, and then her ongoing concern about her everyday family's experience and her child's future.

The clinical material we present demonstrates how we engage a symptomatic toddler while simultaneously addressing his mother's needs for repairing the rupture in her relationship to her child. At the outset, we assume that no matter how a toddler behaves, his behavior has meaning. We hold in our minds that the toddler too has "a mind," no matter how obscured by his symptoms. We start the therapeutic process by "translating" the toddlers' seemingly meaningless actions and sounds into meaningful narratives and comprehensible, reciprocal play. This form of engagement makes "sense out of nonsense" (Bergman, 2007), and not only helps the child arrest his symptomatic withdrawal, but creates a mutual understanding between mother and child of the child's feelings and thoughts. The importance of mindedness has been emphasized in Theory of Mind literature as central for a child's development of a sense of agency and intentionality (Fonagy & Target, 1998).

The analyst's interventions allow a child to make connections, using the analyst's mind, words, and play as a scaffold to signify meaning to himself and his mother. The most important meanings to uncover, in our experience, are those expressing angry and frustrated feelings that seem to have been masked by the child's symptoms. Our experiences have shown that learning to recognize and regulate feelings, especially anger and frustration, is an essential ingredient to synthesizing and integrating emotions with cognition and actions. Helping a child and mother make meaning of the child's behavior is the first step toward recognizing the mind and feelings of others, on the road to having a Theory of Mind. Moreover, knowing what is expected and being able to respond accordingly seems to emanate from processing information and experiences in the playroom, creating a sense of "self" and "other" in myriad, but ultimately predictable, patterns.

We hypothesize that the implicit work of integration that leads to forming a Theory of Mind takes place within the minute-to-minute interactions between analyst and child, and will be illustrated in our case material. In our work with ASD children, we find them to have varying degrees of deficits that seemed to have interfered with development of "Theory of Mind," affecting their capacity to play and pretend (Tustin, 1988) (Baron-Cohen, 1995). Historically, in place of creating an imaginative representational world, our ASD toddlers have engaged in perseverative, concrete tasks with which they are intensely preoccupied. The analyst's consistent work and hovering attention in each hour offsets the ASD child's tendency to continue to fend off stimulation (including his mother's fear of his symptoms) by retreating into stereotypical ASD behaviors. By engaging the child and trying to enter his world, we address primitive symptomatic withdrawal and work towards facilitating safe ways for the ASD toddler to express in play and words his anxiety-ridden feelings and thoughts.

The daily process of scaffolding representative play in turn bolsters development of symbolic functioning in both play and language, including the important step of imaginative play. Ultimately, the dyadic process uses the analyst's playing and labeling of actions and affects as a bridge to the development of a triad of functional connections: between child and analyst, mother and analyst, and child and mother that the child carries from the office to his outside world.

We will present four cases in depth. Two toddlers, Johnny and Corey, had been diagnosed with ASD. Ethan, whose development was "uneven," had been misdiagnosed as ASD, meeting two of the criteria in the details of his presentation. We present him as an example of a child whose uneven development brings similar dilemmas to the family and the analyst as does ASD. Dyadic treatment in these three cases took place with in-depth frequency of 4-times-per week in addition to weekly sessions with the mother or parents. The next section will describe the treatment of Dahlia, a child who was seen in a combination of dyadic work and Reflective Network Therapy in the classroom.

In all three cases in this section, each child received multiple services in addition to dyadic treatment, including speech, language, occupational and physical therapies, and in each case the analyst formed a team to create and maintain coherence. In addition, these families provided additional hours of home-based interventions with caregivers or students who engaged the toddler as many hours as possible in concert with the analytic modality. Johnny, the first of the three boys that will be described began dyadic work at 30 months and by 36 months no longer needed services, although he had an aide in his first months of a nursery program. He entered a mainstream kindergarten at age five. The second child, Corey, began treatment at 25 months and lost the diagnosis by age three and a half, although he needed continuation of speech therapy for another year. Ethan began therapy at age 28 months and was able to enter a mainstream nursery program at 3 years 4 months with some additional classroom supervision.

The three cases of dyadic treatment make for interesting comparisons. ASD symptoms, whatever their cause, become a final common pathway of interrupted communication between a toddler and his parent; often, but not always, empathic and loving connections are obscured or seemingly lost as well. In out cases, Johnny's mother reacted to her child's diagnosis with intense narcissistic pain, seeing the diagnosis as an impossible impediment to her relationship with her child. Feeling stranded, she verbalized her desperation to find any kind of help and empathy for herself. Once dyadic treatment was underway, she was extremely vigilant about the implication of every gesture for her son's future.

Her reaction was, in our experience, more typical than that of Corey's mother, who seemed to take his diagnosis in stride, embrace it, and continue to see him as the loving, cuddly infant he had been. In part, her reaction stemmed from her need to see him as if he were a baby on her knee, attached to her without any hint of need for individuation. Her vigilance came into the treatment by way of questioning the analyst's competence, but never actually questioning the treatment per se. Unlike Johnny's mother, she believed Corey would lose the diagnosis "despite the analyst" while she tested the analyst regularly as a seeming displacement from her anxiety about letting Corey go. Whereas Johnny's mother was more typical in overtly reacting to his symptoms with fear, disappointment, frustration, and remorse, Corey's mother fought the analyst, not the diagnosis! Ethan's mother was quite psychologically minded and bonded with the analyst in an idealizing transferential mode that promoted the success of the treatment.

Like any children on the spectrum, all of our toddlers struggled to some extent not only with their impairment in processing internal stimuli, but also struggled to ward off the ever-present feelings and concerns of their parents, much as these children would need to ward off any kind of overstimulation coming from their environments. The disappointments, hypervigilance, and understandable anxieties about everyday management, as well as concern about her child's future, took its own form with every child/parent dyad we will describe, offering insight into how complex and subtle the mix can be in any individual family. The process material from sessions with these families will portray how the danger of this secondary reaction by a child to his parent's struggle with his symptoms, and separately, with his diagnosis, can disrupt the parent's ability to accept and manage her child's symptoms, even threatening to lead to a downward spiral of developmental disorganization.

Last but not least, we found ourselves being confronted by parents about management of "transitioning" their child under myriad circumstances. Transitions are implicitly invoked in so much of everyday life, but can present enormous difficulty to children with uneven development and ASD due to their inability to process sensory information and parental requests. Often, these children were propelled to either freeze in place or throw a tantrum in order to ward off any change of circumstance or location. Each of the children we describe had his own tool for defending against transitions. Ethan's was the most concrete: he froze, and then grabbed CDs or credit cards, holding on to them for dear life, in order to allow being transitioned from a "known" location to one "unknowable." Corey's mode obscured the problem: he both threw objects and threw himself at his mother, having developed a few routines to maintain bodily contact with her during a transition. Johnny was the only boy who had developed a typical transitional object, his bunny, which he used at home for comfort and for sleep. But, at the outset of therapy, he hadn't been able to communicate his need for his bunny, creating a situation that was, in a way, worse than that of the other two.

In summary, from the point of view of our understanding the developing mind-brain of the ASD toddler, our dyadic play techniques work to establish a foundation of basic trust, and foster, from the neurobiological perspective, the development of mental representations of self and object as well as emotional and cognitive connections that can withstand frustration and limit-setting. We hope to enable the establishment of connections between child and parents that can endure conflict and defense, and promote solid identifications with them. With this newfound ability comes the development of semi-symbolic play and then true symbolic play and language.

CONCLUSION

We will begin our examination of these three children with the presentation of Johnny. As dyadic work with Johnny and his mother shall amply demonstrate, it is useful for a mother to watch her child projecting his emotions—especially hostile, aggressive emotions—into the interactions that are more proto-play than pretend play with the analyst. Johnny's development of affect regulation and discipline began by allowing him to experiment with expressing his aggressive feelings with the active participation of his mother and analyst.

Chapter Two

Johnny

I would like to describe my work with Johnny, who was referred to me at the age of 30 months for symptoms of twirling, gaze aversion, compulsivity, head-banging, temper tantrums, and biting. Johnny had retained a limited vocabulary through speech intervention at 22 months, but was unable to use language to express either his needs or his emotions. Johnny was a fraternal twin, and was the first born of the two. His twin, Tim, was developing on a neurotypical trajectory, making Johnny's symptoms more apparent from their onset. There was no family history of ASD.

Johnny's very early development included babbling, and at his one-year pediatric check-up, it was noted that he made eye contact with his doctor. In many ways, Johnny's cognitive, emotional, and motor development had seemed identical to his brother's. However, while Tim began to say "Mama" and "Dada," and waved goodbye to his parents, Johnny did not. By 15 months, symptoms of gaze aversion and emotional withdrawal were becoming apparent.

When he was about 18 months of age, Johnny's parents noticed a significant change in his behavior. He began twirling behaviors, ignoring his mother, and banging his head on the ground. Additionally, Johnny started to line up his toys in rows, and would lie on the floor, running wheeled toys back and forth at eye level. He seemed to shut out the world around him, and little of his behavior or affect seemed genuine. When angry or upset, Johnny was difficult or impossible to soothe, and he seemed unable to report when he was hungry, thirsty, scared, happy, or upset. Moreover, he would use sing-song speech to imitate his mother. It was exceedingly difficult for Johnny to share his toys with Tim or his mother. He continually sought toys that he could twirl, and his representational play was severely limited. When over-stimulated, he would twirl his body in a methodical fashion. His head-banging and twirling also increased in response to discipline, and he held his fingers in a rigid, stereotypic fashion.

At this point, Johnny's parents sought help from an intervention agency who supplied a therapist with a behavioral approach. Applied Behavior Analysis was put into place starting at about 22 months, which provided Johnny with multiple services of twenty to thirty hours per week. During the subsequent 5 months, Johnny learned his letters, numbers, colors, and vocabulary. Nevertheless, his parents described him at this time as disturbingly "wooden," "robotic," and repetitive in his verbal and emotional expression. Although they saw a slight improvement in his demeanor and engagement with them, he then regressed significantly after the family moved into a new home when he was 28 months of age.

After meeting with Johnny's parents to obtain a history, we decided that I should meet Tim before meeting Johnny, so as to make a comparison and also to determine if Tim needed psychotherapy as a consequence of the family's bias in giving so much attention to Johnny. When I met Johnny, I agreed with the diagnosis of ASD made by his intervention agency. After several consultation sessions with Johnny, we agreed on instituting a treatment plan that included four-times-weekly dyadic therapy with his mother, weekly parental counseling, and continuation of the services he had been receiving, in total about forty hours per week of treatment. His parents and I met with each of his outside therapists as a team on a regular basis and worked to include team members whose therapies complemented a psychoanalytic, developmental perspective.

FROM STEREOTYPIC ACTIONS AND MINDBLINDNESS TO INTRODUCTION OF NARRATIVE MODULES

During our initial consultation, Johnny, who was then 30 months of age, immediately labeled me "Grandma," to which Mother laughed and remarked that indeed, I resembled her mother. Johnny then examined the toys I had laid out and began to run the trucks and cars on the floor. He then lined them up like trains and lay down on the floor, rolling them back and forth and staring at the wheels. At first, I simply labeled his actions, putting into words what he was doing. Then I began to try to identify and label anything that suggested what he might be feeling, watching to see how he responded to my verbalizations by carefully noting his subsequent actions and/or play. For example, Johnny began to bring his favorite toys, Thomas the Tank Engine trains (each of which has a name, two of which share the names of Johnny and his twin) to the office. He repeatedly ran them along the arm of my sofa, putting the trains in many types of danger—crashing, falling, or smashing into other toys. Mysteriously, he would always include in his play some form of "bits" of things, mysteriously calling them "avalanches"—small toys, cracker crumbs, or anything else he could pile up—over which he would run one of his trains or cars. I would take up the narrative, verbalizing the danger that the train was about to encounter, and then gradually introducing an additional train or obstacle to represent his mother's affect. He seemed to respond positively to my explanatory verbalizations, or "mini-narratives," of his mood and wishes by flashing a fleeting smile or darting the occasional look in my direction out of the corner of his eye.

METABOLIZING WHAT THE ANALYST PROVIDED: MODULATING SYMPTOMATIC BEHAVIOR

One of the first acts Johnny initiated was to try to drink my coffee. I had a large mug of coffee sitting on the table, and he sat himself in my chair, picked up the mug, and tried to sip from it. I was so taken by surprise that I simply let him do it, knowing the cup was lukewarm. His mother was extremely anxious that he would spill it and "ruin the carpet," which was the beginning of a two-year conflict over who was in charge of damage control in my office. It undoubtedly resonated with Johnny that I was much more like his father than his mother in my cavalier approach to furnishings, children's behavior, cleanliness, exhibitionism, and brinksmanship. That I stood up to his mother but was simultaneously caring and extremely deferential toward her was not lost on him. I made sure as best I could to not give him the impression that I was going to replace her in his affection. On another early occasion, Johnny and his mother arrived at my office early to a locked door. Johnny responded to this by banging his head on the floor of the hallway outside of my office.

I kept one eye on his mother, observing her frustration, anxiety, fear, and denial of his abilities. As Johnny began to expand his play away from robotic, stereotypic sequences to narrative scenarios, I incorporated my observations of his mother's moods and affects into these figurative, representational sequences. In this type of play, I would try to put Johnny's affect or emotional states into "mini-modules" to bring him out of his autistic shell. Putting his play with toys into words allowed me to continue forging a basic connection with Johnny as well as illuminate for his mother what Johnny might be thinking or feeling. If she didn't know what a particular play sequence was about, I would verbalize what he was doing and make a guess as to what it signified to Johnny. Even if my speculation as to the meaning of his play or verbalization was incorrect, this approach gives the child the experience of someone attempting to understand his mind and his feeling, thereby creating a play space between child and therapist that can be duplicated by the child in his evolving reciprocal relationship with his mother.

Gradually, Johnny began to develop a fledgling sort of "pretend play" with me, using the trains to express his feelings and, on several occasions, spontaneously announcing how he felt. However, Johnny's behavior in my office seemed to alternate between two extremes: sometimes he was rigid and unresponsive; at other times he was playful and cheerful.

During our first month of treatment, I also made several home visits to observe Johnny's interaction with his brother and his early intervention team, comprised of occupational, physical, and speech therapists. I observed he occasionally participated in play with them, though much of his behavior was robotic and he often responded to them with refusal. His behavior worsened as soon as his mother entered the room. It seemed as if Johnny experienced his brother Tim as a barrier to his physical and emotional connection with his mother. Her overt, readily expressed anxiety about being torn between their needs left her helpless to manage the negative affect of either child. If his mother, a helper, and his brother were in the room, Johnny would retreat to the corner of the room with his back to everyone and become absorbed in playing with a toy, not responding to his name. If he was doing something with his brother, it was not reciprocal, and at the slightest sign of Tim being competitive, intrusive, or interfering with what Johnny was doing, Johnny would lash out, run away, or otherwise disrupt the activity.

At 36 months, after six months of our combined treatment plan, Johnny's language and play had grown tremendously. He was able to speak in full sentences, made good eye contact, and could describe his experiences and announce his needs. He expressed a wide range of emotions both verbally and physically. For example, he would spontaneously hug his mother, say he was "mad" or "scared," and acknowledge in words if he did not want to share. Though he did not refer to the future, he was able to describe experiences from his past.

But perhaps the most significant change in Johnny was the development in his play of an elaborate repertoire of narrative situations and representational characters involving family members, cartoon characters, animals, and past experiences, most often using the train "characters" as the basis for his own pretend play. His baby-doll play was semi-symbolic, and he showed identification with the baby as well as the parent, expressing frank rage and aggressive assault on the dolls in one session, and then pretending to be the doll being fed by mommy in the high chair in another. At home he began to engage in rudimentary reciprocal play sessions with Tim and bit or ignored Tim less frequently. He continued to twirl objects when very distressed, but Johnny no longer twirled his body. He had begun to participate in a swimming class, during which he regularly accepted and responded to instructions, happily jumping off of a diving board. Though he became frustrated if not understood when he expressed himself verbally, and continued to need help with his enunciation, Johnny began to appear cognitively and linguistically advanced for his age, as his language use had changed dramatically.

However, when Johnny's aggression was aroused, he often slipped back into his symptomatic behavior, rubbing something on his stomach or trying to gaze at a moving object at eye level. He had occasional temper tantrums, and when angry, he would bang his head on a cupboard or the floor. It seemed as if, after a period of initial intervention, Johnny had become accustomed to what was expected of him, reverting back to his symptomatic behavior when he wanted to tease, test, or manipulate his parents. Johnny's mother, in particular, was manifestly distraught at her son's behavior from the beginning. Through the weekly dyadic therapy, however, she was eventually better able to manage her own aggression and expectations of her son.

BEING DRIVEN CRAZY AND DRIVING OTHERS CRAZY: "CHITTY CHITTY BANG BANG"

The following vignette, when Johnny was 33 months, occurred a number of weeks after the terrorist attacks of September 11, 2001. It illustrates how I worked with Johnny and his mother in dyadic psychotherapy:

> As Johnny and his mother walked into my office, Mother began expressing frustration and annoyance that, over the weekend, Johnny constantly recited the words "chitty chitty bang bang" while running cars, trucks, and airplanes over his stomach and chest, which seemed meaningless to her and his father. Johnny had been watching the Chitty Chitty Bang Bang movie compulsively for some time, and when I asked what the movie was about, she told me that the flying vehicle in the movie (which has windmill rotors that twirl, like Johnny) runs over buildings, crashing into them. As Mother was talking to me, Johnny began reciting "chitty chitty bang bang" over and over, as fast as he could. (I speculated to myself that, with his agitated actions and singsong voice, he appeared to be mirroring her anxiety about his autistic behavior, and perhaps he sensed that his behavior "drives her crazy." He might also have been expressing his feeling that their anxiety about his diagnosis drives *him* crazy. After 9/11, there was still much anxiety about the "twin towers" and possible continued terrorist attacks, and children with processing difficulties easily conflate fear of external events with fear of their own aggression and retaliation.) Johnny asked me for potato chips, and as I was getting them, he reached for a toy train and ran it back and forth on the table, reciting, "chitty chitty bang bang." His mother looked very irritated and frustrated. By this point, he and I both knew that this stereotypic behavior signaled his distress with his mother, his knowledge of her disappointment in him and in me because he was still symptomatic, her despair that he was irreparably damaged, and his way of blocking her out and driving her crazy at the same time—his punishment of her for all past and current "crimes"—all of which I had verbalized at one time or another over the previous few months. I picked up a toy

train and joined his play by imitating him, saying "chitty chitty bang bang" and mirroring his tone of voice, which grabbed his attention; he looked straight at me, making direct eye contact. Johnny then tried to stand on my block box, which I saw as a hint, and so, I took out blocks. Speculating about the content of the movie, a vehicle crashing into towers, I built a tower for him to knock down, handing him a large block. He appeared reluctant at first, averting his gaze, his body language seeming as if he were checking out how acceptable it would be to be that aggressive; I thus took the initiative and knocked the tower down myself, saying: "The tower crashed! It was so scary!" I then rebuilt the tower, and this time he imitated me, using the large block to knock it down. This play became reciprocal, as we then took turns knocking down towers. He then expanded the play, and seemingly acknowledged the connection to the movie's action, by reciting "chitty chitty bang bang" as we played. He then went into the toy cupboard, pulling out the book about Spot the dog hiding from his mother. I said, "You are worried that Mommy will be angry at you for crashing the towers." He looked up, directly into my face, and stared at me. "Yes," he said. After eating a few more potato chips (which served as a form of refueling and soothing), he picked up a school bus and, pretending it was a plane, called it "chitty chitty bang bang" while gleefully making it crash into the blocks. I said, playfully, "Watch out, the tower is going to crash!" He then yelled at me, full of excitement, "What are you doing in there?" I responded, "I am working in here!" Following his lead, I leant down to put my body in the middle of the block towers he had crashed, and again he crashed the bus into the tower of blocks in which I more or less was lying. I said, "Oh, no, I am dead!" to which he replied, "I want chips!" Then, while we had more potato chips together, I told him, "The twin towers were knocked down, and everyone in New York was scared—Mom, Dad, me, and you, but it is all over now." At that, Johnny looked straight at his mother, making full eye contact, as if looking for confirmation, leading me to say, "Your mother will protect you, and hug you, and take care of you, and so will your dad." As I was talking to him (but, in fact, to both of them), Johnny maintained eye contact, his mother smiled at him, and then hugged him. And, then, he picked up the bus and replayed the crashing scenario multiple times. (Turning passive into active gives a child control over the titration of aggressive feelings.) Johnny then elaborated on the play by toppling over on my head as I pretended to be buried in the blocks. I continued to moan about how scary it was to have the tower crashing on me. He then picked up a block as if to hit me, which clearly scared his mother, who looked shocked. I could see that he was teasing, and said, "Johnny wants to scare you, Mom, the way that he has been scared!" After asking for juice, he took out the ABC book and sat in his mother's lap, letting her read new words to him, his affect quite calm and peaceful (this situation being a much more typical type of refueling), making consistent eye contact.

"WHAT ARE YOU DOING IN THERE, PINOCCHIO?": REPRESENTING LAYERS OF ANXIETY TO JOHNNY AND HIS MOTHER

> As they got ready to leave, cleaning up the blocks into the box, Johnny stuck a long triangle block into a pile of blocks, half-burying it, and said, "What are you doing in there, Pinocchio?" and then, "The water is scary!" and "He is lost!" He then yelled, "Pinocchio! Where are you?" Following his lead, I said: "Pinocchio is made of wood, like the blocks, and he is lost, and scared. He has lost his mommy and daddy and is all alone in the water, inside the whale." Johnny continued to call out, "Pinocchio, where are you?" and tried to bury his hand in the box. I then said, "Your hand is buried in the rubble!" and he indicated that he wanted me to bury both his hands in the blocks. As I did so, he kept calling to Pinocchio, wrapped up in this play, while his mother watched, flabbergasted, marveling that he hadn't seen the tape of Pinocchio for at least two weeks. (Earlier, she had protested that he couldn't possibly have known anything about 9/11.)

DEVELOPMENTAL SCAFFOLDING: SENSE MAKING AND MAKING SENSE

In this session, by closely following Johnny's mood, words, and behavior; by joining him through mirroring him and then labeling the process, I was able to put into words his many layers of anxiety—that is, about his parents' anxieties about 9/11 and the fate of Johnny's autism, about his mother's frustration with him in my office, his own anxiety about his "scary" feelings, his wishes to hurt his mother, his father, and Tim, his fears of losing body parts, of driving his mother away, of driving his mother crazy, and of being physically separated from his mother, as well as his wishes to be hugged and comforted—all of which he had heretofore been unable to express, avoiding body contact with his mother and refusing to look at her. We thus translated his symptoms of preservative recitation of "chitty chitty bang bang" into meaningful communication; making his experiences understandable brought his mother relief from her anxiety about his condition and freed her up in the moment to respond to his needs and physically comfort him.

EVIDENCE JOHNNY SEES HIMSELF THROUGH HIS MOTHER'S EYES

Another interesting point concerning this session is Johnny's reference to Pinocchio—an uncanny response to his mother's frequent complaint that Johnny was "wooden." Hence, was he beginning to represent himself through introjection of her, by naming his hand "Pinocchio," whom he knew from the movie to be a wooden boy? This play also shows the transition from concrete play to semi-symbolic play, in using his hand to represent something hidden. Johnny's running of the cars back and forth over his belly also illustrates a typical defense we see in toddlers—turning passive into active, controlling the movement of the car out of a need to control external stimuli of noise, light, sound, and conversation, as well as his anxiety about separations.

THE SYMBOLIC LANGUAGE OF SEPARATION: "POOPY CAKES," "MONSTERS," AND "WILLIES"

Johnny's transitional object was a stuffed toy bunny, which became a source of consternation to both parents, particularly his father. They would argue about whether or not he was allowed to take his bunny, for example, out of the house, to a restaurant, or later, to nursery school. It embarrassed his father that his son would be seen sucking his thumb and rubbing his bunny against his nose in public. Also, at various points in time, Johnny had been punished by different people in the household by taking his bunny away, as that was the only recourse action which would guarantee keeping him in line, although his mother stated she felt "terribly guilty" every time she did it herself.

As our work on these aspects of separation/aggression progressed, Johnny began to show us for the first time that he was aware of his genital area. In his play, he also started to become curious about the toilet. We spent a lot of session time in the bathroom, flushing toilet paper and snack food, and, as I began to playact the disappearance of objects by saying "bye-bye" to them, he labeled them "poopy cakes" and tried to drink the toilet water. Next, he began asking where those things were going! In subsequent play, he then picked up his bunny and examined it between its legs, looking for its "poop hole." This play then led to his negotiating with his mother for her to leave the session (for the first time) to get him a snack.

Knowing that Tim actively played with his penis in front of Johnny (who reportedly had avoided ever touching himself), I thus begin to transition my remarks from interpreting separation from Mother to addressing his fear of losing his "willy" (as the family referred to his penis) if he were to touch it, looking for the developmental thrust—that which was missing from his play or verbalizations, but was nonetheless expected at his age. Thus, when he ran his cars on the hard edge of the sofa, I took this to mean that the hard car on the hard edge might be serving as a reassurance against castration as well as mastery over his fear of losing Mother, that is, the treacherous mother became the treacherous edge. I also told him when he ran his cars on his stomach that he was reassuring himself that he still had his "willy" without having to touch it, and that he was pretending that the car is attached to his stomach—that the car could be hard without having to worry about losing it. After this was fully interpreted, he dashed to his mother, who was sitting on the sofa, and ran his car over her body, starting at the bottom of her foot, moving up her leg, over her abdomen, around the outside of her breast to her neck, and then over the top of her head. At this point, in front of Johnny, his mother told me that he had run his hand up her body and over her breast at home, but explained this in a defensive tone, saying that she was wearing loose clothing, so the action was less obvious than that which had just occurred. This remark showed, I felt, her denial of his interest in her body.

Then, amazingly, Johnny picked up a girl doll and said, "Her willy is gone." Surprised, I thought to myself that he couldn't possibly have been able to think about where it *went*. That would have seemed too cognitively advanced—too high a level of abstraction compared to his other abilities with language and abstract thought. Yet I decided to take a flyer, so to speak, and while he was rolling a tractor on top of a car and avoiding me, I said, "The boy baby is scared of seeing that the girl's willy is gone." He stood and came over to where I was sitting with the dolls, looked at the doll, and said, again, "Her willy is gone!" Then, to my amazement, he asked, "Where did it go?" He peered into the space between her legs, looked at the hole there, touched it, and asked, "Did it go inside?" He then picked up a cupcake and ate it with pleasure and absorption.

"GRANDMA CRY!": THE IMAGINATION ACTION LANGUAGE OF ANGRY AND SCARED FEELINGS

When Johnny was nearly 3 years old, 5 months into the treatment, separations were dealt with by variations on play of hide-and-seek. Prompted by his mother's report of Johnny's behavior on the family's Christmas trip, I pretended to be Johnny and enacted her report. I complained, "I miss you, and you are locking me out," and, then, "I want to go home. I don't like Hawaii anymore . . . I swam there, but then I threw myself on the ground and cried, and now I want to come back!" Looking me directly in the eyes by way of confirmation, Johnny said, "Leave again!"

> In response to Johnny beginning an hour by lying on the floor and kicking my toy cupboard, Mother chastised him—at which point he tried to bite me, saying, "Grandma, cry!" I told him that the monster (a theme established during previous sessions) was in my office, and that we had to feed him potato chips. Again, he told me to cry, and then said that "Mommy is a monster, too." I suggested that we feed Mommy some chips, but he replied "No!" in a stubborn manner. I offered raisins or Cheerios, but he didn't respond, instead going to the couch and laying behind the cushions, a location he had previously referred to as a "cave." This time, however, he didn't label the "cave." I suggested that perhaps he was hiding as he remembers when his mother left him at 18 months

> to go away, and I asked him, "Where did she go?" I also told him that he was behaving at that point in the same way as he did when she left. He then emerged from the cushions, stood up, and said, while looking at the door, that there was a television there, and "on the television there were many, many butterflies—mother and baby butterflies, and kings, the bumblebees were the kings, and they were scary. The butterflies went down to the water, they were falling in, and then the little butterflies, and then the bees followed as well." He continued this strange, lucid narrative, prompting his mother to ask if it was from a video. I asked him if it was from a dream. He was insistent on trying to get his mother to understand the butterfly sequence; his mother later remembered that when the family was in Hawaii, there was a bush Johnny had seen with many bees living in it. At the end of the story, he labeled it a dream, repeating that the baby butterflies were scared of their mothers.

In expressing his angry feelings like a 2-year-old (by kicking the cabinet) Johnny enacted his "monstrous" feelings, instructing me to "cry," showing a change in his handling of his aggression and attempting to redirect us into interactive play. He associated his mother's absence (at 18 months) with the baby butterflies' fear, both of the mother butterflies and of the scary king bumblebees, possibly representative of his father. The fact that the butterflies (the mothers, then the babies, then the bees) went down to the water "as if they were falling in" shows Johnny's simultaneous desire and hesitation to follow his mother in her absence; it seems that he is unable to trust her ability not to "fall in." The "many, many" butterflies may be a reference to his being one of many—a reference to his twin-ness. From the perspective of his emotional growth, this "dream" signifies his ability to express his thoughts, fears, and needs in a way that Mother can understand, and therefore be prepared to offer him protection—for example, the butterflies are afraid of the bees, and the baby butterflies are scared of the mothers. In psychodynamic lingo, we are seeing in status nascendi the emergence of Johnny's capacity to symbolize, in rudimentary fashion, the emotional states of others (Fonagy's "Theory of Mind" or "mentalization") as part of the process of development of reciprocity between mother and child. The internalization of Mother's response to his fears, for example, is a step in the sequence that allows the object's affects to be introjected in such a way as to solidify healthy ego functioning.

In the ensuing weeks, Johnny's play became more layered, and seemed to demonstrate an emerging struggle to form representations of what he saw in the external world and what he felt inside. As mentioned before, Johnny had been engaging in sequences of play wherein he would first pretend to cry, and then pretend to be a monster that made me and Mother cry. I labeled the pretend play with the monster as "scary," and would fend the monster off with my potato chips. During one important session, I said to Johnny, "I guess you feel like a monster when you don't want to share with Tim."

Mother then interjected that Johnny had bitten his twin a lot over that past weekend, after which Johnny announced that he and his bunny were going to go and hide in the cave. (I wondered if the cave represents that he is ashamed of not sharing, or if he wants to hide from retaliation.) Next he played going out the door, and saying "what's going on here?" I repeated that he felt as though he were being made to share with me, like Tim, and remembered feeling like a monster as a baby, having to share mommy and being angry about it.

Similarly, the separation play expanded to include his anxiety about losing his poop and his mother down the toilet drain, and to frank castration anxiety and interest in the genital difference. For example, Johnny picked up a naked rubber boy doll, pulled its legs apart, and then set it on the edge of the play box. At that very moment, his mother noticed that Johnny was "having a poop!" So, I said, "This boy is pooping on edge of the box, and we have to look for the toilet," and then, pretending to be the doll, I began to cry, "I don't want to poop; I'm afraid to lose it in the pot; it's too scary;" etc. In response, Johnny picked up a red stick and poked it through the holes in my chair. "Oh," I said, "losing your poop makes you think you might be losing your willy down the poop hole. No wonder you don't want to poop on the toilet! I had better keep my diaper on so I don't lose my willy!" Mother then said, "Tim and Johnny talked a lot about willies last night—Johnny watched Tim push back his foreskin," and wondered aloud if perhaps Johnny had never seen the tip of his penis. Johnny immediately exclaimed, "Cocoon! Cocoon!" to which I replied, "Ah, it looked like it was coming out of a cocoon!"

Typically, a developing child would be working through rapprochement while simultaneously being toilet trained, and hence confronting inside-and-outside, self-and-other differentiation, and castration anxiety (for boys), as well as mastering his or her aggression stirred up by the demand for good behavior, developing reciprocal means with his or her parents to cope with conflicts about hanging on and letting go, and struggling with sexual difference. Analytic work, unlike natural development, tends to force more sequential processing than does everyday life, where demands for appropriate behavior supersede any awareness of the underlying developmental thrust. The analyst's job is to put into words what might otherwise be left unspoken, and moreover, to make sense of the play by being more specific, or more artificial, or more arbitrary. One is constantly choosing individual routes on encountering forks in the road, addressing one developmental line and leaving another developmental line behind.

Accordingly, as the sessions progressed, Johnny's play became highly complex as he struggled simultaneously with these developmental issues that were no longer sequential. For example, Johnny seemed to be struggling simultaneously and quite suddenly with both his urinary and anal functions, with castration anxiety, and with genital difference, all while still working through his relationship to his mother and her narcissistic vulnerability at seeing him in any way as symptomatic—she continued to remain very worried that he would stay "autistic" for life.

So, for example, in another session, Johnny told me that he woke up with a "frog in [his] diaper" and then pretended to be a frog under his coat, which made me guess that he had likely woken up with an erection that frightened him, which I then interpreted.

He had observed that his brother was not afraid of playing with his own penis, and I wondered if Johnny was struggling with their difference. On one occasion, his mother had brought him in while also carrying a bag containing two cupcakes: one for Johnny, and one to take home to Tim. After eating his own cupcake, Johnny insisted on eating the second one as well. I took this opportunity to make a reconstructive interpretation—that he would like to be an only child. I wondered out loud if perhaps he remembered thinking that he was an only child when he was very little. (I was hypothesizing that, between twelve and eighteen months, his inability to process the world around him might have interfered with his forming a mental representation of his twin, further confounding the mother-child separation/individuation subphases.) In response, Johnny made a face that made him look exactly like his twin, whom he does not ordinarily resemble in facial features or expression. In this context, Johnny finally began to sleep through the night.

Transitioning from semi-symbolic toilet play, Johnny began to express anal, phallic, and separation conflicts through symbolic play, first by covering blocks with paper, then by using a bang-a-ball-toy and little people. He returned to projecting his feelings about his conflicts onto me, "making me cry" while he played at separation, loss, and anxiety about missing or broken people and body parts. Soon after, he began to show an expanded repertoire of affects. For example, he showed surprise, acted out his fears of certain toys, and then asked me to draw faces for him, where he showed an interest in assembling the parts of a face for the first time.

"SHE'S KILLING ALL THE CHILDREN": IMAGINATIVE PLAY WITH HIS BODY AND BI-GENDER IDENTITY

By age three and four months, Johnny was regularly talking with Tim about "willies falling off," especially when bathing. In subsequent sessions, he examined the holes of two girl Fisher-Price dolls and said, "They have willies." He also began to play with himself, rubbing his groin with one hand underneath his body while stretched out on my analytic couch. Projecting his fear of retaliation onto me, he had me pretend to be a monster and threw balls at me, saying, "The monsters are biting the willies!" During this play, he bit me twice. His mother was appalled. I explained that we had to distinguish between his being fragile (which he wasn't), and naughty (which he was), and that discipline would not hurt him, but would instead help decrease his fear of fantasy retaliation. This was the beginning of my dialogue with Johnny's mother about how much she feared that saying "no" to Johnny would cause him to regress to an autistic state. Thus, she was unwittingly letting him "get away with murder" at home. His awareness of his preferential treatment made him increasingly guilty toward Tim, and besides not helping Johnny's ego development, I pointed out that this caused his twin to suffer as well.

In my session with the parents that evening, they told me about their struggle to develop a system of time-outs that worked for both boys, especially because Johnny was being regularly provoked by Tim and then assaulting him in retaliation; they, meanwhile, were glad Johnny was "whacking" Tim. While telling this to me, Johnny's father laughed and said, "I wish I could do that!" His mother smiled in agreement. It was clear to me that Johnny was expressing his parents' anger toward Tim as well as their own toward each other, controlling Johnny in order to control their own aggression.

Johnny's mother was terrified of the boys' turning out like her brothers, who sought danger and disasters growing up in Hawaii—there were toes bitten off by sharks, crashed planes and cars, and so forth. His father was more cavalier and often referred to his wife as a "ninny." The following session is an example of my work with Johnny at about age 3 and a 1/2 that shows the process as well as my thoughts in the moment of the session. In this session, Johnny takes pleasure in his urinary prowess, his phallic exhibitionism and in teasing his mother, uses projection of his bad boy behavior onto me as a method of managing his fear of retaliation, and incorporates his response to her fear of his following in her brothers' footsteps. It also shows her fear of her inability to control her own behavior, her depression (whether situational or not, I could not say), and Johnny's identification with her unconscious anxieties—as well as how it potentially interfered with the development of his own superego. (My thoughts are given in brackets, which I am providing in order to inform the reader of the way they guided my interventions in the session. They were not spoken.)

> Johnny came into the office and yelled, "Bad boy!" at me. In response, I said, "Oh, Grandma's a bad boy!" He said, "Grandma—bad boy—cry!" [Projective identification, evidence of evolving mental representation of the other.] He then took two male Fisher-Price figures from their box, looked into the holes and said, "They have willies." He started twirling a car on his chest, which kept dropping off. [I wondered if this represented a twirling penis.] He subsequently went for the scissors, making an attempt to cut his shirt, and did indeed make a little cut in it. [Displacement of penis activity to his chest; things are

falling off his chest and twirling around on his chest. I think, "this play is extension of conversation and play at home."] With this in mind, when Johnny said, for the third time, "Grandma is a bad boy, cry!" I went to my chair, sat down, and started to cry as though I was having a time out. I called out, "Mommy, Mommy, can I come out?" His mother asked him, "Can Grandma come out?" Johnny said "no," appearing thrilled, and made direct eye contact with me. I continued to cry like Sarah Bernhardt. Mother kept asking Johnny if I could come out, and Johnny went to her purse to look for Bunny. [Bunny represents a threatened punishment from parents—taking it away—here, conflated with castration anxiety?] I cried that I wanted Bunny. He sat on Bunny so I couldn't get it for about five minutes. He then found the car he called "chitty chitty bang bang" and ran it on the couch, being "symptomatic." Mother leaned over to see if he made poop and announced that she was going to the bathroom to change him. I overheard Johnny referring to gender differences (for the first time), saying that Alec was a boy, and Katherine was a girl. Also Mother made a negative, anxious comment about how, being in the bathroom, he might have to do water play. [This constitutes a threat to her, and her anxiety about water play is obvious to Johnny.] And so, he proceeded to do the very thing she feared—becoming boisterous, filling cups with water and floating a boat in the sink, drinking the water, saying "wee-wee," and using the toys and water to represent symbolically drinking "wee." [I could feel his mother's ambivalence and anxiety while he was doing this—her negative reaction to me letting him play this way mixed with her wish for him to get the help he needs.] He then spilled water over the back of sink, onto the floor. Mother made a sour expression and asked if it was okay. I let it happen without answering to see how she would handle the situation. When Mother told him he couldn't fill up cups anymore, Johnny moved away from the big sink to the toy sink where he made artistic arrangements with various colored objects in pots. He took nesting blocks, filled them with water, made them go "wee-wee," and took them apart and tried to crush them like crushed chips in the toy sink. He began to show an inward gaze, much like when he was "making poop." With a much livelier affect, he said something about the blocks being knocked down by Charlie, a book character. He took the nesting blocks out of the sink and put them on his chest [phallic representation], and the water dripped down the front of chest [phallic displacement upward], while I was talking about his pleasure in making the blocks go wee-wee, even though Mommy didn't like it. He grinned very happily, and by this time, he was totally wet. But soon, Mother's anxiety about his being wet made him get whiny [he regressed]. She took his shirt off. I decided to explain to Mother what I was observing—how frightened she was of aggression. Right in front of Johnny, still in the bathroom, I told her that when he had just then been at the sink, he understood that she was anxious about his spilling water on my floor, and had moved to the toy sink, to play artistically in a symbolic way that he knew was acceptable to her. His peeing and pooping play would be healthy if organized in a symbolic fashion, but in fact it represented, at that moment, his unconscious anxiety about things breaking off and being lost. With the artistic play, he reconstituted these feelings, showing that he could move back and forth from regressive spilling (as brought on by castration anxiety) to symbolic play, and then was able to go back to actual phallic play. I said that if she were

> this frightened of his aggression, he wouldn't be able to express his aggression in a healthy way. Meanwhile, Johnny had started pulling toilet paper off of its roll, dropping it in the toilet, and saying that he wanted to make "poopy cakes." We have, of course, done this before. He did his usual play of making "poopy cakes" in the toilet, with his shirt still off. Mother and I conversed about her transposition of his normal aggression into something acceptable, like a sport—throwing balls, for example, or playing in the tub. She whispered to me that she was afraid that Johnny would become a mass murderer, and that she had a dream the previous night in which he threw himself out a window. [She recognized that this was in association to her being frightened of his aggression.] I said the dream she cited along with the confession of her fear for Johnny's future had nothing to do with mass murderers, but was instead about him getting in trouble and being in danger. I told her that she would have to discuss the dream with her own therapist—she was clearly terrified of her own aggression. [I refrained from telling her that her dream represents her anger at her children for being difficult and her consequent wish to throw them out the window.] I suggested that she join a group to discuss parenting.

GOING FORWARD

The following several vignettes present sections of sessions demonstrating the evolution of various aspects of Johnny's cognitive and emotional development—although this is far from a complete survey, these examples illustrate the main thrust of the work that progressed over the next two years. Specifically, these samples illustrate our focus on limit-setting and superego development, the vicissitudes of his anal, urinary, phallic, and oedipal conflicts, and the development of symbolic, metaphorical play that sprung up later in the course of his treatment, at about age 4-1/2 years.

Focusing on supporting limit-setting can be an important part of work with this age group, as illustrated by the following scene. On one occasion at age 3-1/4 years, when his behavior was naughty—his hands were sticky with chocolate, and his mother, obviously frustrated with him, wanted him to wash them—I chose to address his naughtiness rather than letting him play at making messes. I introduced a game where I pretended to have my hands talking to each other, one being a "sticky monster" and the other the admonisher. I used one hand to tell the other hand that it had to go to jail, and hiding the naughty hand behind my back, I said, "The sticky monster was very naughty and is going to jail!" to which Johnny asked, "He's having a time out?" I said, "Yes," and he immediately exclaimed, "Do it again!" After several repetitions of this, Johnny told me to lie on the couch and go to sleep. He then took his mother to hide with him in a corner, and announced, "Me and Mommy came to scare you!" Using his hands, he pretended to be the sticky monster, saying, "He tried to bite me while I was sleeping!" Then he went back to the corner and played very quietly with his mother, so as not to wake me up.

An interesting aspect of Johnny's development during this period of time was the way in which he integrated his bowel movement into our work during our sessions. Typically, he would move his bowels and would then try to avoid being changed by his mother or caregiver until the session was over. Even after he was trained, he continued to use our session and my bathroom as the primary time and location for his bowel movements. He had occasional urinary and bowel accidents at home and school, and brought into the play his humiliation at messing himself, as well as his fear that his teacher or mother would be mad at him.

Johnny's play showed that he connected his messing himself to his anxiety about genital difference, as if being chastised by mother or me could lead to being turned into a girl. For example, while pushing his foreskin back during his bath, he asked his mother where her "willy" was. She responded, "I have a vagina." Johnny asked her if she was "X," a character that can transform from boy to girl, and then asked if he was a boy because he had a "willy." Meanwhile, he continued to use the anal mode to express aggression—when he was angry with someone, he would pretend to "poop on [his or her] head" and would laugh gleefully. He enjoyed his sadistic fantasies, and in developing more control over his aggression and his fear of retaliation from his brother and mother, he made another developmental thrust forward, shifting to more phallic themes of stealing, falling, and breaking things. This included pretending to make cars and trains fall into pools of sharks, which he would often follow up with a defensive game of connecting a mommy, daddy, and baby train together and making them follow each other around the office.

In the context of this play, I finally understood the consistent, perseverative action of his running cars over piles of potato chips or "bits" of things and calling them "avalanches." This time, he piled a group of toy children on top of each other and ran the "mommy" truck over the pile of children figures, killing all of the children in the pile. Thereafter, killing and being killed became very prominent themes.

Also during this same period, at which point Johnny was nearly 3 years and 6 months old, whenever I addressed his mother as "Mommy" during our play, he would angrily interject, "She is my mommy, not yours!" I would then correct myself and refer to her as "Mrs. L." Each time I would "slip up" in this fashion, he would correct me.

Subsequently, the normative negative oedipal themes emerged, wherein he pretended to be female, or me, or his mother, expressing his preference for the color pink, trying to put on my lipstick in the office, and trying at home to put on Mother's clothes and steal his female cousin's necklaces. Part of his struggle with his identifications was expressed in his curiosity and concern about why he was in therapy, how his mother felt about it, and why his brother was not seeing me as well, which were reflected in his play with creating avalanches, crashes, and rescues. In his phallic excitement and fear of retaliation, I found myself unable to parse out who I was in the transference—as we began to play hockey with our blocks, he could not tolerate my scoring a point. He began to ask me personal questions for the first time, cognitively taking a leap to understanding that I was also a real person. He asked me if my 25-year-old assistant was my mother, and, "Where do you live? You don't live here? You live somewhere else? You are going home?"

When he asked explicitly why he had a "play doctor" and Tim did not, I made him a chart on which I listed his and his brother's differences and similarities.

Another developmental step, from around age 3-3/4 years, shows his identification with his mother as the love object of his father. For example, he locked me out of the bathroom so that he could make lunch for his children. He hid his bunny under his shirt, saying that it was in his tummy, and then pretended to put his children to bed. He then yelled for me to pretend that I "try to take [his] babies away" from him. "Why?" I asked. "You're not a good listener!" he yelled back. [This is an imitation of his nanny.] Then, worried about possible retaliation, he said, "I'm kidding! Let's go skiing!" [Here, he is imitating his father.] When his mother then tried to find out why he had been angry with his father, he yelled, "I'm very mad 'cause you took away my bunnies!" [For some time at this point, he had repeatedly expressed his desire to make babies with Daddy.]

This layered scenario also seems to show Johnny's identification with his father's prohibitions about being a baby, especially those concerning carrying his bunny outside the house, but also wanting to please Daddy by being like him (i.e., a skier), resolved at the moment by becoming the father of the babies.

More and more, as he turned 4, I found myself approaching the crossroads of supporting either his regression or his superego development. For example, when he would make a mess on my table with water and paints, he might refer to cleaning up. Following his hint, I would then suggest that we clean up, strengthening and solidifying the restraints of his impulses rather than pursuing them. Then, seemingly overnight, Johnny showed an apparently discontinuous developmental shift—from playing semi-symbolically with cars and trains, he turned our play into the story of *Harry Potter*, externalizing all of his "bad" impulses onto the Slytherin (the "bad boys" in the novel). The story then became the context for all of the themes he was exploring in our work—based around the concept that boy figures had girlfriends. He paired up with the heroine, Hermione, and played out his oedipal rivalry—his competition with his twin and with Father. He also began to use the chess set, using the kings and queens and their children as families—he created sets of good parents and bad parents, who may or may not have been protecting or rescuing their children, but who nonetheless fought against each other. He explored where babies come from through our pretending to make secret potions.

In addition, he demonstrated a new defense of reaction formation against wanting to be an only child through play wherein he imagined that a mommy bird had laid many eggs in a nest that a monster bird tried to rob. He became panicky about going to sleep and being awoken by monsters, and insisted that I make a home visit to talk to their "ghost" and tell it not to come into his bedroom. When I arrived, the boys were in their pajamas and robes, and we had quite a conversation about the ghost. They started hitting each other, playing "monkey in the middle," and then Johnny got on top of Tim, at Tim's request, to put his nose in Tim's anus. On reflection, there had been some hint of this in sessions where Johnny played derivatives of wanting to seduce Father, particularly in laying on and rubbing father's stomach, and in earlier sessions where he was pregnant with Bunny. I suggested therapy for Tim. (Tim was quite masochistic and sadistic in a sly, manipulative way, but mostly provoked Johnny to attack him and then tattled on Johnny. I also learned that Johnny had put his finger in Tim's rectum, as well as his own.)

Johnny's mode of aggression in his new play was mixed—it was sometimes anal and sometimes phallic; for example, he played that bombs hit Harry Potter's castle, knocked it down, and broke it to pieces. "Everything breaked and the castle breaked and the magical wand breaked!" he had said. Thus, he announced that both his phallic instrument and its object, the castle of the Mother, were doomed! In response to his own fantasy, he became scared, and proceeded to pretend that he had to hide in a cubby that we had made—and then sent me into the cubby to sleep, thus making me the baby he had created with his mother. He then took out our "war" toys and shot at me, turning me into the pregnant mother.

His subsequent play was a fascinating condensation of two co-existent themes—our work on separation, where we continued to explore and reconstruct his annihilation anxiety from the pre-verbal period, during which he could not process his fear of loss and abandonment, and his new fear of intercourse, typically expressed in children of this age as "dying." We had this play sequence after his attempts to play out his penetration fantasies and anxieties; in the context of playing that his mother had left on vacation, while playing at the toy sink, the following transpired:

> "All the children died," said Johnny. "First Theodora, then Johnny . . . then all the children died [they were "drowning" in the sink]. . . . Oh no, now they all died. Oh no! Help, help, help!" [At this point, he had three more "children" die, all while two watched; he then put them into the boat in the sink.] "None of the children are left; they're all dead," I observed. "Now two more children

> are dying!" exclaimed Johnny, throwing them into the sink. "Ann and Charles died," he said, "now he died . . . everybody died!" "Now they've all died?" I asked. Johnny sang, "Die, die, die, they all died, now they're all dead, now there's no more children." "And when their mommy comes back from vacation, they'll all be dead!" I said.

He not only played that the children were lost, but that I was sent to jail, as the queen, for this crime. Meanwhile, he anxiously grabbed at his penis a number of times, demonstrating that not only could Mother be banished, but that the penis was in danger as well. In this context, he developed a symptom of gnawing at his index finger so that the skin around his nail looks, in his words, "flayed." He would later tell me that a ghost was threatening him and his soccer team when the coach would turn away, and that gnawing at his finger kept the ghost at bay. "All their skin comes off and they turn into skeletons, and dinosaur bones, and somebody comes and eats them," he had said. Meanwhile, he regularly threatened me, as a Slytherin, with the threat that "I will cut off your willy!"

With an increase in scenes of kings and queens involved in baby-making, and then endangering those babies, he showed further anxious genital arousal, touching and rubbing himself against the furniture. He created a solution in his play—to set traps for the Slytherins, sending snakes to guard the black holes. This play alternated with his use of the Harry Potter story to enact his conflicts via two camps, in which he pretended to be himself, fighting his twin. (Much later, they would be conceived of as a team, sometimes protecting each other against a common enemy.)

At age 4 years and 9 months, Johnny was faced with a new challenge—to apply to a mainstream private school for kindergarten. In their nursery school, he had been placed in a class with his twin, who watched him like a hawk and reported on Johnny to Mother, constantly comparing the two. The theme of his brother's spying and "tattling" on him in school had been contributing to our Slytherin story line, and Johnny retaliated in our play by spying on the enemy boys and then demolishing them. In reality, however, it turned out that despite Mother's intense anxiety that Johnny would not be able to tolerate taking the ERB, he outclassed his twin with scores in the ninety-ninth percentile in the verbal section, and in the ninety-fifth percentile in overall performance. He also outshined Tim at every school interview.

The following process notes detail some of the recurring, pertinent themes during this period in time, just before a two-week vacation:

> He made a circle of his children, the Fisher-Price figurines, within a circle of parents. We were protecting the children so that they could keep the telephones (which they had stolen from me) to themselves. Then, he began to search for a piece of paper from the previous session, on which I had originally written the word "CAT" for him, but then at his insistence had crossed out

> "CAT" and written "DOG" beneath it. I procured this paper and showed it to him, but he insisted that there was an additional paper, one which somehow only had "CAT" written on it. Poignantly, he had a total meltdown because I couldn't produce this imagined piece of paper, instead only being able to show him the one which had "DOG" on it as well. He became stuck on the idea that there was a second piece of paper, and nothing Mother or I could say or do could move him from his mounting hysteria that we were wrong. He then sought to soothe himself by requesting his bunny.

This situation not only seemed to be an association to the theme of unprotective parents, but also a reversal, in his conception that his mother and I were defective and had stolen the piece of paper from him. This did seem to me to be a nidus for understanding how concrete such children can be when "symptomatic," and condensed his sense of being both "castrated" and "autistic." Meanwhile, the bunny clearly provided soothing that he couldn't get from me or his mother, because we had been the "bad guys." In the transference, I had, for the moment, become the hypervigilant mother who kept searching for evidence in his behavior that he was "still autistic," humiliating him, wounding his narcissism.

After addressing how the bunny soothed him, and how mother and I had hurt his feelings, I linked his meltdown to the upcoming vacation (thinking also of the telephone play, which was new). After a bit, he turned the play back to our previous "castration anxiety play" by talking about the little children having "willies" stolen from them. He was then quite calm, and asked to eat his cupcake. However, his play association was most remarkable, and spoke to the regression to the time of "autistic" derailment—he demanded to sit in an old wooden high chair that is used for dolls. I had to tell him that he couldn't sit in it because it was rickety, and I was afraid, because of his size, that not only wouldn't he fit, but that he could break it further. He then sat in my chair, but complained that he felt "lost" because he was too big for the high chair, highlighting the multiple determination of the idea of "lost" in his fantasies. At the end of the hour, he kept insisting he wanted to take my telephone home with him, so I gave him my business card with my telephone number on it.

In the next session, Johnny tried to convince me to let him stay overnight in my office to protect him from the monsters. He verbalized that Sally, his nanny, wouldn't let him take home the saltine crackers he ate in my office, because his father would disapprove.

DEVELOPING A SYMBOLIC LANGUAGE FOR CASTRATION AND PHALLIC IDENTITY

At age 5, he told me that the punishment for the Slytherin would be that their wands were to be taken away from them, a metaphor for the fact that Johnny's father had robbed me of my power by forbidding me to feed him saltines in my office. He then had us play that Hermione gets hurt and is sent off to the hospital. He announced that he, Harry, was taking away all the wands from the boys and proceeded to put them in my lap (I was sitting cross-legged on the floor next to him). He put the wands in the space between my legs, calling it the "crosshatch," then put the children there as well, making a "magical" sound while giving them "crystals," which he acted out by dumping a pile of Pez in the middle of my lap. He made a clearing for the Pez in my lap, held up the dispenser, and proclaimed, "You are going to have this—it has a secret compartment, and it will make you powerful!" Then, he activated a light on the top of the Pez dispenser, so at that point I had a flashing phallic rod on top of all the children in my crotch. Johnny proceeded to make several grandiose remarks about its power and glory, took the children out from my "crosshatch," and tossed them against the wall of the castle in handfuls. His mother, trying to control her laughter, excused herself to go to the bathroom.

Following this scene, Johnny plotted that the children were attacked by sharks, tarantulas, crocodiles, and snakes, and told me, "You are crazy!" He also told me that women "are crazy" because they put things "in the wrong hole," all while he played at poking things into holes, or while we talked about wands being "trapped" and/or bitten off. He then pretended to fly off on a broomstick, like Harry, suffering a broken leg from falling off. "Girls have holes, boys have willies!" he announced, while simultaneously yelling that he is afraid of being "trapped!" [This is apparently a reference to vagina dentata.] "Your weenie is going to break," he told me.

As we worked through the themes that were interwoven throughout his play, evidence of an emerging "ego ideal" resonated with the threat of oedipal retribution, on both the narcissistic and phallic level. For example, Johnny started to play "God," hiding behind my chair, scaring me, and then announcing "I am God!" "Is this true in real life?" he would ask about various things, wondering if he could be protected by God. He played at stuffing soldiers, robots, balls, and other objects into the tubes of the bang-a-ball toy, referring to the tubes as "dungeons," and designated the pink ball as the present for the "winner." This play seemed to me to be highly suggestive of making anal babies, and his pronouncement that, "He [the pink ball] will never be alive again—he's closed into the dungeon," was very suggestive of claustrophobia.

This play also pointed to his questioning his gender identity as another variation of an attempt at oedipal resolution, that is, not to "have me," but to "be" me, a phallic mother. Evidence of his reaching for narcissistic omnipotence seems to conflate here with the complex process of identifying with me both in the transference and as a new object—variously the "good mother," the "phallic mother," "Mother God," and the castrating mother.

At age 5-3/4 years, the twins entered their new school, a mainstream kindergarten, where they were placed in separate classrooms. As both boys struggled with the challenges of social acceptance and being separated, the manifest content of our sessions turned somewhat to the question of "who is in, and who is out," conflated with play that was also clearly primal scene-based, which included a lot of "spying." Johnny created an elaborate Lego clubhouse in a block castle where the all of children were paired up in couples, and he had a particular girlfriend whose identity was kept a secret from his brother. The couples attended a disco dance that excluded the parents. "I want to come [to the office] seven days a week," he announced to me. "I want to live here!"

In addition, he sprinkled his play with phallic activity, using a large piece of puzzle to cover a hole so that a snake could not enter; other times, the giant snake was guarding the hole. During this period, he ate a hamburger for the first time; meanwhile, in our play, giants descended on the children to eat parts of their bodies, and the robots were often broken into pieces. As school progressed, he developed acute anxiety about his performance and conflict about creating a separate identity—and having separate friends—from his twin, which took the form of holding in his urine and ultimately wetting himself in school. Thus, his conflicts about his urinary sadism and phallic excitement were defended against by symptom-formation, not only expressing these repressed wishes by wetting, but which had the secondary gain of being committed "by accident," thus soliciting empathy instead of retaliation.

INTERNALIZATION: THE OUTCOME OF "PARTICIPATORY APPROPRIATION" OF THE ANALYST'S DEVELOPMENTAL SCAFFOLDING

As I sensed that Johnny was on the edge of latency, with consolidation alternating with fantasy elaboration, his struggles with the superego issues of ego ideal, internalization of controls, omnipotence, and retaliation became increasingly prominent in a number of ways.

First, his question of whether his parents or I were the ones "in charge" became dramatically real when Johnny's father challenged me openly to not feed him crackers during our sessions. Johnny became very resistant to coming because I was not standing up to his father over what I deemed "cracker fever." I found myself struggling with the appropriate response, sometimes giving him the crackers in spite of his parents' wishes, but mostly complying. We both were confused about whether I could not stand up to his parents or would not do so, but it was clear that he wondered what had happened to my magic powers. Most likely, I was not only losing my omnipotence with Johnny, but with his parents as well. He was struggling with his disappointment in me—his knowledge that I was a real person who is not perfect, but also that I was a maternal/paternal transference object who was no longer idealized. In his play, our magic password became "police."

Second, Johnny manifestly tested his parents and his brother at home, expressing the question of who was in charge of his body and mind, that is, parental control versus the internalized superego control over his conflicts. For example, when he began to wet himself, his father clearly viewed this behavior as shameful and infantile. Johnny told me, "My father said he will take me to the hospital if I wet my pants again!"

Third, in our sessions, Johnny continued to project evidence of his struggles with superego resolution by making me be the policeman, right up until the last hour of our last session. It was clear that he believed that if I were the police, he could remain in a state of impulsivity and excitement.

Fourth, as evidence of his aggression toward me escalated, I came to think that he needed to be angry with me in order to leave. For example, while pretending to hide in the clubhouse to "protect the children," exhibiting reaction formation and identification with the aggressor-teacher-parents, he became very rude to me, making it clear that I couldn't say anything "right." He then drew a picture of me, crossed it out, and tested me by insisting on taking the jacks home with him in order to "have power over wanting to kill" me while also obviously magically holding on to me. "I am going to pray that you die before I have to come back!" he told me. In the next session, he mischievously grabbed a box of toothpicks and stuck them vertically into my chair, trying to get me to sit on them! In the following session, he drew a black heart and wrote "I HAT[e] YOU" on it, and drew a picture of me crying, then cut off my head, and cut my heart in half. He finally announced that I had "poo" on my face.

Lastly, I saw that he was in dire conflict about having succeeded in achieving somcthing in analysis that was denied his twin, with emphasis here on "success neurosis": our sessions became flooded with wishes that it would be Tim's turn to see me, and "couldn't [I] straighten Tim out?" Still, however, the rivalry was expressed in anxiety that I would thus come to love Tim more, or that I would find Tim to be more of a boy than Johnny, who still clung to his color preference of pink. For example, while complaining that he was still very angry at me about the "cracker veto," Johnny announced, "I am very angry at my mother!" and ran to my chair, grabbed my lipstick from the sideboard, and applied it all over his mouth, creating a clown-size smear, all the while grinning with fear and excitement. This evidence of sexual identity confusion in the face of fear of oedipal and sibling retaliation was also demonstrated in the subsequent session in which he played at poisoning the children with lipstick, drowning them, and then having the doctor resurrect them by doing "surgery on them to fix them." At the end of this particular hour, he yelled at me on his way out, manifestly because I wouldn't give him any crackers, saying, "You are awful!" and "You are dreadful!" and "You are sexy!"

TRIAL CONSOLIDATION AND SEPARATION FROM AMBIVALENTLY LOVED OTHERS

As we edged toward a planned termination for June of that year, Johnny became technical in conversation with me for the first time, which I felt to be evidence of emergent latency, by saying "I asked you," in reference to a previous topic of discussion. And, indeed, he truly wanted the answers—again, signaling latency: the answers to where babies came from, and other sexual secrets.

His ambivalence about ending the analysis was expressed in his making me a large paper medal which said, "1st Prize for hating Sherkow." He then proceeded to make a profound mess of my office, dumping everything he could get his hands on onto the floor. Subsequently, partly in reaction formation to having to fend for himself, he created a new kind of play in which there were two armies, the good army and the bad army, but in which his brother had become his partner. "Do partners kill each other?" he asked me, playing that the two of them were standing against their parents. Then, he had me make a medal for his twin in Tim's favorite color, blue. Johnny ultimately decided that he could not kill his partner. This, I felt, was the resolution of his rivalry with his twin—because he needed his brother to be his partner; they needed each other to fight their parents.

Just before the upcoming Christmas vacation, Johnny's play became more organized around the theme of testing me, while increasingly relying on the twin-ness for support against the powerful monster—me. The testing took the form of more dumping of anything he could manage to dump, gleefully prancing around the mess. He demanded that I make two paper ribbons, as we had done in an earlier session, to pin on him and his brother, on which he advertised how much he hated me (thus making believe that his twin joined him in this). Around this time, as I was wondering how severe the dumping behavior would get, he began both to continue to act very proud of the mess, but also to ask me if I was going to call the police. For a number of sessions, I responded in the negative while attempting to interpret his behavior. Finally, when at my wits' end, I responded to his query by saying,

"Yes, I am gong to call the police!" and reaching for the phone. He abruptly stopped dumping, and that entirely ended the behavior. Soon thereafter, he expressed anxiety and had nightmares concerning again leaving for Hawaii, and fears about swimming in the ocean "with the sharks." In his play, having recently visited the Egyptian wing of the Metropolitan Museum of Art, he became preoccupied with mummies and artifacts, and I remembered that I had something in my bin that he could use as a magic token—the bird head of an Egyptian god. He announced, happily, that he was going to take it on vacation to protect him.

During the last months of treatment, Johnny's play reflected, increasingly, his concerns about integrating with his classmates, making friends, and competing with and/or identifying with his brother. His play behavior—featuring exclusive clubhouses, Egyptian tombs, and hieroglyphics—continued to move in the direction of latency, with primal scene and family romance themes now embedded in his interest in Egypt, magic tricks, invisibility, vortexes, and especially masturbatory derivatives.

In our last session, he pretended to be his brother, holed up in a fortress that I, cast in the role of Johnny (and specifically identified as a "spoiled brat"), could not penetrate. He made it clear that he, playing Tim, didn't have to go to a "feelings doctor," but did have a hole in his heart, a double entendre on the then months-long theme of "broken hearts." In the very last moment of the session, as he was walking out the door, he left singing, "I'm gonna kill you, baby," to which I replied, "I love you too. . . . Bye!"

CONCLUSION

It is hoped that this case description illustrates two significant dimensions of our work with young children on the spectrum. First, we believe it demonstrates that it is possible, using psychoanalytically informed dyadic treatment as part of a global intervention, for a child who clearly demonstrates signs of ASD to later lose the diagnosis. Second, it also demonstrates the confluence of factors Johnny faced in overcoming his neurofunctional deficits while at the same time struggling to master the age-appropriate tasks of ordinary development in a toddler about to turn three. We worked in therapy to address the breadth of object relations, separation-individuation subphases, and development of ego and superego all the while keeping in mind the impact of his neurofunctional differences on his ability to keep up with his twin, a special challenge. Alongside his twin's working toward mastery of psychosexual stage-related drive derivatives and evolving super-ego development, Johnny suffered from the inevitable sibling battles for dominance, his ASD diagnosis playing a significant role in his competition for attention with his twin.

Johnny illustrated in his early relationship with his mother the extent to which her attempts to love and soothe him were apparently perceived as disruptive rather than otherwise. In addition, he enacted reconstructions of painful scenarios arising from the historical evidence that Johnny's symptoms become apparent just as he was approaching the process of separation-individuation, likely conflating timewise his loss of the ability to communicate with intense separation anxiety and clingy, demanding behavior. From Johnny's perspective, watching his twin cling to his mother, and seemingly unable to approach her for comfort himself, one could imagine might have exacerbated his withdrawal; but we didn't need to imagine. Johnny's play revealed, in exquisite detail, his feelings about a mother bird "having too many birds in her nest," and his conflict about throwing away his rivals, a condensation of his fear of being eliminated because of his ASD deficits and his intense rivalry.

My observations of Johnny's mother also showed one variation of the impact of an ASD diagnosis on a parent, who understandably reacted with a multitude of affects in the course of Johnny's first years, including fear, anxiety, disappointment, frustration, and remorse. Multiple iterations of Johnny's play at "the mother is killing all of the children!" and his avalanche play, where almost from the first sessions he ran a car (it turned out to be the "Mother" car) over the piles of chips/children, eventually were verbalized. Also from the beginning, it was apparent how both mother and child participated in warding off the other, until we reached the session in which Johnny and his mother could both accept his aggression, displaced onto the "twin tower," which in turn revealed his understanding, all along, that she thought of him as "wooden." This session began the process of reestablishing an empathic connection between them.

We believe the disorder contributes to the child's perceiving his mother, in particular, as an inadequate developmental object, which works against his developmental strivings, contributing to his frequent expressions of humiliation, rage, and frustration. From early on during the treatment, I speculated that Johnny could not internalize his parents as fully developed objects because of his neurobiological deficits. I further speculated that there were mechanistic differences to be found in aspects of his brain functioning that had likely impacted his ability to process cognitive with emotional stimuli at a synaptic level, a supposition supported by the medical literature on this topic (Helt et al., 2008). Given this scenario, Johnny's brain development would have prevented him from being able to process his experience of his parents as complex objects, in contrast to his neurotypical twin. This in turn would have prompted him to perceive and internalize his experience of his parents as exaggerations of part-objects, that is, angry, and scared of him and his diagnosis. Later in the treatment, after his development appeared to be more "on track," I speculate that he continued to struggle, nonetheless, with internalizing his parents as developmental objects because his mother continued to represent herself to him as being terrified of the possibility that he would retreat into symptoms of autism if she disciplined him. Moreover, Mother certainly continued to represent herself to Johnny as being frightened and unable to shake the impact of his original diagnosis, or "deficit."

From the point of view of our understanding of the developing mind-brain of the toddler, dyadic therapy works to establish a foundation of basic trust, and foster, from the neurobiological perspective, the development of mental representations of self and object as well as emotional and cognitive connections that can withstand frustration and limit-setting. In other words, it promotes the establishment of connections that can endure conflict and defense, especially in building solid identifications with the parents.

Working with Johnny points to the advantage of beginning treatment as early as possible, especially before age 3. The earlier the intervention, the more likely the toddler will remain verbal and begin to attain the development of cognitive and affective connections, expediting the goal of preventing the exacerbation of—and possibly reversing—the underlying neurological abnormalities (Dawson, 2008).

A final thought: in my experience, children use songs to develop language and to regulate affect. I often introduce something new to a child by singing it rather than saying it, even if I use the same melody over and over ("we make mu-sic, we make mu-sic," which is to the tune of "Frere Jacques," and which is the only tune I can sing). This allows the child to withstand the stimuli of putting a negative feeling into words, furthering the emergence of language. Does the accompanying music act as a grounding or organizing force coming from a neurobiological mechanism for the development of language?

Chapter Three

Corey

OVERVIEW

My work with Corey and his mother, Mrs. A, was significantly different from my work with Johnny and his parents in several ways. Although Corey had received speech and occupational therapies from the time he was diagnosed, at 18 months, he had not responded, due to his overall temperament, lack of focus, and absence of modeling of language between himself and his parents. They were not aware, most likely, that he was not ambiently absorbing the structure of language. Johnny, by contrast, had acquired words through speech therapy, and although he did not use them to communicate, he was also exposed to his twin's verbal connection to his parents. Corey overall was much more babyish. Mrs. A's personality also seemed to have much more influence on our work and seemed to have contributed to shaping Corey's symptoms and course of his recovery.

Early on I observed that Mrs. A seemed to have reinforced Corey's neurofunctional biological failure to individuate in his second year of life by virtue of overvaluing their closeness. Beneath the surface, we gradually learned how threatened she was that Corey might become a separate individual, including his being a boy. Mrs. A's fear of Corey's separation/individuation spilled over into our first months of therapy.

In our introduction, we set forth the hypothesis that some ASD toddlers fail to make sufficient neural connections for formation of progressive cognitive and thus language structures, and this in turn appears to shape their ability to "read" themselves. They are equally unable to use words and gestures to make their mothers aware of their emotions or needs. In addition these children appear functionally unable to internalize a schema of representing their mother's actions and feelings toward them, with consequent disruption in basic trust, well-being, and the building blocks of ultimate self-regulation.

We saw, with Johnny, how much both Johnny and his mother had pulled away from each other during the year between the emergence of Johnny's first symptoms and his entrance into treatment, with increasing layers of distrust, miscommunication, and ultimately aversive behaviors on both of their parts. Corey's first two years were quite different. He and his mother remained affectionate and "bonded." Mrs. A appeared to feel gratified by Corey's continued utter dependence on her during his early toddler phase, when he more "typically" would have been practicing separating from her and gaining some competencies that would gradually help him become independent.

In addition Mrs. A seemed challenged by the need to help Corey self-regulate and manage his aggression. For a toddler beginning to walk at the end of his first year of life, the biological forces that propel him into action need to be harnessed by a combination of parental controls and the internalization, mutual mirroring, and reciprocal scaffolding between parent and child. Limit-setting and containment of her toddler act as necessary reassurances of her presence and interest in his safety. Corey's mother was an excitable, charming, and somewhat grandiose woman who seemed to manage her competitive feelings through a narcissistic investment in being "right," and, by extension, through denial of the fragility of her toddler on the move.

Corey was a rambunctious toddler who had over-developed the mechanism of throwing. He threw himself on his mother and on and off the furniture. He loved to randomly throw objects. This behavior raised the question of its meaning with regard to intentionality or implicit approval of his mother as she consistently ignored it. Indeed, Mrs. A's tendency to attribute Corey's difficulties to external sources seemed to impede her ability to better understand both Corey and his experience. His mother's conflicts in this sphere impacted Corey's own conflicts and interacted with and reinforced his ASD vulnerabilities, regularly enhancing his overall symptoms, at least as we saw them in the office.

In part I was able to help Mrs. A and Corey by offering intensive attention to both of them in dyadic "play" as the first step toward helping each of them better understand the other. I was concerned from the outset that Corey had shown little capacity during our consultation sessions to internalize my attempts to help him represent his needs and feelings. I also quickly ascertained his mother's diminished ability to relate cause-and-effect, to facilitate "anticipations" and transitions, and to allow for belief systems other than her own. Ultimately this dynamic would appear in the transference through Mrs. A's fear, anxiety, and anger that my ideas and mindset would take over, shaping our relationship by virtue of her hypervigilance about my actions and her hovering intrusiveness with regard to what I was thinking.

Nonetheless Mrs. A embraced my recommendation: Corey would receive a 30- to 40-hour per week engagement in the cognitive and emotional world by combining four days a week of dyadic therapy in my office with an individual session with Mrs. A, in addition to daily hours with a trained, home-based adjunctive therapist. From the outset, my goals for treatment were to help Corey develop language, self-regulation, and the capacity for categorical learning. I sought to understand what seemed, at first, to be Corey's meaningless behavior, and I also endeavored to help Mrs. A understand how her parenting impacted her son.

INTRODUCTION TO CASE MATERIAL

Corey was an adorable, lively, brown-haired, brown-eyed 25-month-old toddler when his mother consulted me to evaluate him for ASD. Mrs. A reported that Corey had not developed babbling or "pointing," although he would use a gesture to indicate forbidden foods he seemed to crave. Indeed, because Mrs. A was careful to provide Corey with a gluten- and dairy-free diet, he mischievously devised ways to climb onto the kitchen counter and help himself, which indicated his ability both to exercise agency and to "read" his mother's prohibitions in at least one area. He was affectionate with his mother, using her body or grabbing her hair when in distress, but he made no social gestures such as "hi" or "bye." Neither did he have a name for his mother or father. He made only fleeting eye-contact and was unresponsive to his name, requests, or directions, and he demonstrated poor social and interactional skills. He was interested in toys only for their mechanical properties but not for pretend or imaginary play.

From early infancy Corey had been a somewhat low-tone baby who drooled persistently, which had continued to the time of the referral. Although he was always "cuddly" with his mother, he was averse to being held by his father or other relatives, including his full-time nanny. When at 18 months Corey's pediatrician documented "an expressive and receptive language disorder, as well as failure to demonstrate joint attention, consistent with the diagnosis of Autism Spectrum Disorder," Corey's mother was referred to an Early Intervention Agency for comprehensive services. These included speech and language therapy, occupational therapy, sensory-motor stimulation treatment, "floor-time" therapy, and physical therapy. His mother attempted to enroll him in a playgroup to promote social skills, but the director felt he was too immature and lacking social awareness and instead referred him to the author for intensive psychodynamic treatment.

My first encounter with Mrs. A's tendency to be vague and ambiguous with recounting details or forming a narrative occurred when I tried to form a developmental picture through taking Corey's history. I struggled to learn how or whether evidence of Corey's early symptoms might have impacted Mrs. A's relationship with him. It was also difficult to form a clear picture of Corey's relationship with his father, who had separated from Mrs. A when Corey was about 8 months old, although he visited regularly and frequently and was very supportive of Corey and his therapy.

Mrs. A's overt congeniality and air of compliance in our initial meetings alternated early on with shifts in her tone. For example, during her second consultation she asked, "What do you mean by 'aggression'? Why do you focus so much on aggression in describing how you work with toddlers?" Later she confided, "I was impressed that you answered my challenging question without flinching!" This communication was emblematic of what I came to see as an ambivalently dependent transference to me, clinging to me even as she seemed to be invested in questioning and even purposefully obfuscating the nature of my work with Corey.

My immediate impression, borne out throughout the treatment, was that Mrs. A believed Corey was "only hers." She often dressed them in identical outfits, and she conveyed that only she was capable of being in tune with Corey, reading his needs and enabling him as he (they) wished. This included allowing him to share her bed at will, to bathe with her, or to wander in and out of the bathroom when she was using it. In this respect, Mrs. A displayed another variation on the theme of her inability to see Corey as a child capable of having a mind of his own and who would recognize the differences between his and his mother's bodies or be affected by seeing her using the toilet. Corey's neurobiological unevenness in development, wherein he was compromised in the ability to form his own thoughts and initiate his own actions, reinforced a conflation of Corey's innate inability to process language with his mother's struggle at seeing him as "separate" and letting him individuate. This was evident, as will be demonstrated, in the early phase of treatment when Corey seemed to show no understanding of "inner and outer," of "self and other," or of "self versus Mother." He thus mirrored his mother's blurring of the boundaries between them.

Another significant aspect of what appeared to be her denial of his "otherness" was her refusal to allow me to mention his penis in the office and presumably not to let him acknowledge his "penis" in general, which contributed to his gender confusion throughout his pre-oedipal phase of development. In short, who is the boy? How can he be like his father? Can she allow a triangle to develop or emerge?

CLINICAL MATERIAL

Mrs. A suggested that my first meeting with Corey take place in their home so that he could become accustomed to me. There I could also observe him interact with his various specialists and with his father. My first impression of Corey was that he was physically very appealing, wearing long bangs that nearly covered his eyes and lent him a "unisex" appearance. He made no eye-contact or babbling sounds, seemed not to notice that I was there, and was constantly on the move. He did not seem to be responsive to anything that was said to him or about him in his presence, and made multiple attempts to gesture toward and climb onto the counter to procure foods that were limited or forbidden, including dog food.

However, one could not say that he could engage consistently in "pointing" as a form of communication. He showed spontaneous affection toward his mother and had a particular gestural game with her in which he would present his elbow to her for a kiss. He often seemed to spontaneously throw himself at her to hug her. By contrast, and less randomly, he threw himself at her or grabbed her hair when he seemed to be in distress, including but not limited to the infrequent times when his mother said "no" to him. He made no observable social gestures, such as "bye," nor did he acknowledge my presence in any way I could identify. He made, at most, fleeting eye-contact with his mother. He was unresponsive to his name, requests, or directions from her during the visit. He altogether confirmed her report that he showed poor social and interactional skills in general.

Although the apartment was abundantly full of toys and apparatus for physical activity, Corey seemed interested in toys only for their mechanical properties, and although he was lively, he swatted his toys, showing no evidence of imaginary play. Throughout the visit, Mrs. A either talked "at" Corey or spoke for him, unable to facilitate his engagements with either playthings or with me. "Show Dr. Sherkow" was a frequent, but useless, directive.

Over the course of the next weeks, I also observed Corey with each of his special education therapists, and I noted that he was unfocused, showing no evidence of affective investment in the therapist or the tasks at hand but rather performing actions by rote. In all, it was hard to even imagine a meaning behind most of Corey's behaviors, with one exception. He wordlessly demonstrated his love for jumping on his mother's bed after acrobatically climbing onto her stationary bicycle, which was positioned near a picture-window, and walking on the windowsill beside it.

When I questioned Mrs. A, as tactfully as possible, whether she had ever thought permitting such behavior at home might lead to Corey's reproducing it elsewhere, she seemed surprised I would ask. It brought to mind an almost identical mother/child pair I had known, in which the mother denied that she had entertained any such concern. Both mothers struck me as having permitted their normal common sense to be distorted by a combination of feelings that had evolved from managing their ASD toddlers. First, they were happy that their sons had "an interest" that was clearly expressed, and thus wanted to reward the boys' speaking for themselves, regardless of the consequences of the child's wishes. Second, they feared temper tantrums, which were particularly severe when an outright request was denied. Third, they feared the very act of denying their son's wishes would cause a regression to an avoidant/aversive stance. Finally, they feared hurting their sons' feelings. These lapses in judgment, I observed, were not lost on their children, who understood the bending of "rules," as I later discovered when they were able to enact their relationships with their mothers in their play.

FIRST OFFICE SESSION

In his first session in my office, Corey cheerfully bounded into the room ahead of his mother. Without glancing at me, he picked up, dropped, and threw toys in a perseverative manner. He made neither speech sounds nor eye-contact with me or with his mother, drooled regularly, and generally behaved throughout the first hour as though I were not in the room. His mother and I sat in the middle of the playroom to observe him.

For my part I wanted to see if I could identify and label any discrete feelings or intention other than throwing. Unlike a neurotypical toddler, Corey showed no overt evidence that he was in a "new" situation with a new person. His affect varied. At one moment he was lackadaisical, floppy, and unengaged and the next he threw himself quite suddenly into his mother's lap. He alternated between these behaviors without any seeming connection to his picking up and dropping of toys. Sometimes he would also give his mother a hug or present his elbow to be kissed, as she had previously described to me.

I have found that the technique of imitating or even literally mirroring (copying) an ASD child's behavior, words, or actions invariably engages a child, possibly through the element of surprise. It also helps a child know immediately that the analyst is inviting the child to be understood. In beginning to try to engage Corey, I imitated him where possible, followed him, and picked up and dropped toys. "Look how that toy dropped on the floor!" I said. Corey, seeming nearly "mind-less," paid no attention. I continued, "Corey seems to be enjoying throwing the toys—look how they fly!" When he would throw himself into his mother's lap, I labeled that as well, trying to put into words whatever "intentions" I observed in him. Between observations I wondered aloud about the effect his actions might have on himself, his mother, and me.

MAKING MEANING

Very quickly, in the course of our early work together, Mrs. A joined in labeling and vocalizing about Corey, and we tried our best to guess what might be motivating him and to read his "mind" and emotions, especially his hostility. She worked with me in each session, on the hypothesis that Corey's throwing represented a way to express aggression that was not "meaningless" even though it was not visibly connected to an object. If there was any "intentionality" it seemed he was directing most of his hostility to the toys. The few moments of direct expression of hostility (e.g., pulling his mother's hair or flopping wildly into her lap) seemed disconnected at this point in the therapy from any sense of its meaning.

Interestingly, however, in the first months of treatment there were also moments Corey seemed to show more "agency" and intentionality, in contrast to the seemingly random contact described above with toys and his mother's lap. He would use a toy in a scenario or action that seemed as if it could be representational. In one example of representational behavior, he put a small mother-doll on a toy bed and then put the bed and doll into a dollhouse. In another moment, he sent little cars sequentially down the ramp of a toy garage in what seemed like very organized play. When these moments of seeming intentional, representational play occurred, his mother and I would gently try to expand the play scenario by putting his actions into words. However, when his mother and I spontaneously added sound effects to these moments of doll or car play, Corey turned away or threw the toys. By not responding to, and indeed turning away from, efforts his mother or I made toward "joint attention," Corey made us wonder whether what seemed like "representational" play was merely random.

In the absence of any semi-symbolic behavior, either language or gestural, that indicated thoughts accompanying his actions, it was very hard to know what meaning to make of Corey's actions and his responses to his mother and me. Because I approach children like Corey with the premise that everything has meaning, as a way to understand their unique subjectivity, I assumed there was also meaning in Corey's strange response to our attempts to join him. I could not make sense of Corey behaving as though our "joining" or "understanding" him interrupted his "play" and drove him away. But even such unsatisfactory explanations invoke "intentionality." One possibility was that there was no intentionality in the "play behavior" but that he mimicked play sequences that were part of his speech or occupational therapy. I had witnessed his therapists using toys in order to elicit speech or particular skills. Perhaps those play sequences were stereotypic and had no intrinsic meaning to him, or he possibly used them for comfort. If that were so, it still suggested a connection being made in a mental representational system, even if it was one that neither mother nor I could identify.

THE EARLY AGGRESSION

Corey frequently went into his stroller-bag to find snacks and drinks, and my office would quickly become a total wreck of popcorn, spilled water, and small toys. Mrs. A's attitude was nonchalant about his messing and I accepted his need to mess but did not understand it. It was difficult to determine whether Corey was expressing any object-related aggression in his behavior or whether Mrs. A was indirectly expressing negative feelings toward me by her casual attitude toward the mess, in contrast to Johnny's mother, who was always worried about Johnny destroying my office. Another possibility was that Mrs. A's tolerance for mess reflected her comfort with me.

Another early sign of aggression was evident to me whenever Mrs. A became annoyed or upset with Corey in the office for demanding food, or whenever she would bring in an anecdote about something upsetting to her. He would then make aggressive physical contact with her: he threw himself at her, rubbed himself on her, put his elbow in her face to "kiss his elbow," signaled to her to "eat tummy," or would climb on top of the couch or table to leap on her. In general Mrs. A seemed very relaxed about Corey's actions, and her demeanor, in contrast with my experience with other mothers, was the opposite of hypervigilant about the nature, meaning, or prognostication of his behavior in my office.

A pivotal session took place two months into Corey's treatment, immediately after the A's returned from a weeklong trip. I will present the session almost in its entirety, given how dense Corey's emotions and interactions were with me in the course of this one hour. I begin with evidence of how disorganizing separations from me could be for both Corey and his mother.

Mrs. A and Corey arrived in a state of unfocused, anxious activity. Although I assumed Corey was reacting to the separation as though it were "my fault," I wasn't so cognizant of its impact on Mrs. A until the following episode at the very beginning of the hour: Corey, being more particularly unfocused than usual, went in a few seconds' time from banging a waiting-room chair to sliding cars down the ramp of the toy garage, to finally hunting in my cupboard for something to eat, grabbing and shoveling a whole box of raisins into this mouth. In those same few seconds, Corey's mother, in a very garbled fashion, tried to explain the health value of yellow raisins as compared to more common brown ones, praising me for having yellow raisins at the same time as she was criticizing me for having raisins at all. In addition, she criticized Corey for gobbling his food instead of eating in a more civilized manner.

I intuited that in this scenario Mrs. A was trying to communicate her inability to discipline Corey herself, as this disclosure had been accompanied by the expectation that I would be able to read her mind about what and how much Corey was allowed to eat. It had not yet occurred to me to what extent mother, and Corey as a reflection of mother, was struggling with the hiatus. I proceeded to say, "Corey, your mother will let you eat the raisins as long as you eat them without gobbling and instead eat them one by one." I felt my intervention succeeded both in organizing her thoughts and so provided a clear message to Corey about her expectations of him while also implicitly addressing her not-so-subtle projection onto me of her own conflicts, which made Corey feel she was criticizing me and thus putting him into a state of conflict in relation to me. Corey's response was a very clear indication of experiencing my intervention as organizing, because he suddenly began focused play in which he lined up a long string of cars to send them down the ramp. Each time he did, he said, "one by one," imitating my remark about how to eat the raisins, repeating this organized sequence several times. Corey's repetition of my words was noteworthy. While his babbling had increased, he still had few syllables and no syllable yet to refer to his mother.

After the multiple repetitions with the cars, Corey surprised me. He picked up a dollhouse cradle and bed, squeezed them together, and put a small mommy-doll in the cradle. Not knowing if his choice of a mommy-doll was intentional, and thinking about "joining him," I offered to put a baby doll in another, identical cradle. At first, he seemed to allow this intervention, rocking the cradle for a few seconds, but then he threw the baby away and put the mommy-doll in the baby's cradle to rock it. I tried to puzzle out the meaning of this play. Was the use of the specific dolls intentional or random? Was he reacting to my attempt to join him as an intrusion and thus throwing my "intrusion" away, or was he expressing something, perhaps related to conflicts around autonomy, in making the baby disappear? Did squeezing the cradle and bed together have a meaning? Was it a semi-symbolic representation of squeezing Mommy or a by-product of separation/merger conflicts with mother?

Regardless, in the next part of the session I pursued labeling everything he did, using the word "Mommy" as often as feasible. The intentionality behind his cradle play seemed proved by the play scenario which followed. He alternately put the mommy-doll in the bed and then in the cradle, rocking her each time, and letting his mother and me sing lullabies along with his "bedtime play." After several minutes, he added a new sequence in which he put the mother doll in a chair, prompting me to add a table next to it. His mother interjected, "Feed the Mommy raisins at the table?" He threw away the table, seeming to show that he understood her question and responded with a hostile rejection. As with the earlier play, I couldn't discern if he was "throwing away" the act of intrusion or rejecting her as a "feeding object."

This play sequence was followed by his rummaging through the toys, picking a plastic elephant. When I approached him with the elephant, he pushed it/me away, grabbed several markers, and stood, looking as though he wanted a piece of paper. While I looked for drawing paper, he took a big bite of marker, streaking his face. Bewildered by his mother's apparent calm, and not realizing in the moment that Corey was trying to express anger at me, I walked him to the bathroom saying, "I guess you wanted to bite something!" Mrs. A remained passively in the background. Was she also angry at me?

Then, as I tried to wash his face, Corey bit my finger!

"I see, Corey, you want to bite *me*!" As I spoke, he bit me again, although not hard. I went on, "I know you are angry at me, but you can bite this." I offered him toy toast. He stared straight at me for a few seconds and, for the first time, made and maintained eye-contact.

I realized Corey struggled with angry feelings at me for having let him go on vacation. By the time Corey was roused to using his teeth to express his anger, his emotions were crystal clear. In retrospect, his mother and I had been struggling to make sense of expressions of aggression so distorted and defensive they were unrecognizable as object-directed. Once I put his anger into words, Corey became organized enough to establish and maintain eye-contact. I was helping him tolerate, although not yet manage, his aggressive feelings toward me, which had been overwhelming and disorganizing to him.

Once I addressed Corey's feelings about separating from me, I was able to make more sense out of the remainder of the session. After speaking to him about biting me, he took long wooden blocks and built a tower, allowing me to help. We then knocked the tower down. This was all a first for him and was followed by multiple turns, building and knocking down block structures we built together, our first truly reciprocal and representational play. This seemed to be confirmation of the value to him of having identified his negative feelings in the context of seeing his feelings would not destroy me. Moreover, the building and knocking down of towers enacted, in semi-symbolic play, the feelings he was experiencing. This made it possible for him to have positive and negative feelings in turn and so to recover.

Gradually Corey moved from the building play to another new action in which he intensively focused on trying to balance two blocks on top of one. He then tried to build a tower out of three blocks on a tabletop he could barely reach. When his attempt failed, he threw the blocks. I guessed that the three blocks represented the three of us and that failing led to "throwing me and his mother away" and, conversely, also represented his feeling we had thrown him away. I felt surer of making an intervention in saying, "You are throwing the blocks away because they wouldn't do what you wanted!" Corey's response amazed me: he picked up some raisins off of the floor and used them to play hide and seek, a further representation of his struggle to master separation. I said so. "You are playing hide and seek with the raisins!" At that, Corey turned and left the office altogether, engendering another interpretation from me. "Bye-Bye, Corey, you went on vacation!" And then, "Here you are again!" He giggled as he repeated this play numerous times.

I noticed in this latter play Corey was suddenly stringing three- and four-word utterances together and approximating the word "raisin." Although he still had no "M" sound, he had a "Da" and some guttural sounds. I found it significant that language emerged in several moments during intense interchanges in this session, suggesting the break in sessions played a role in organizing a cognitive/emotional representation of me and/or intense feelings of aggression connected to me, which led to a developmental leap.

EMERGING CAPACITY FOR SYMBOLIC REPRESENTATION

The next day Corey demonstrated interest in alphabet blocks for the first time. He allowed me to label the letters: C for Corey, M for Mom, D for Dad, and S for Dr. S. His play association was to invent a "train" using plastic blocks on which he balanced a plastic elephant, pushing this "train" on actual train tracks. He allowed me to add two little trains, ran them briefly on the tracks, and then undid the "train." He then took the elephant off the train, took apart the two cars I had put together, and found a crib-like cart into which he put the elephant. I said, "The elephant is in his crib!" He stared at me, giggled, and gleefully repeated this sequence multiple times.

Again I offered a play elaboration, asking, "Should we give the elephant a bottle?" guessing the elephant represented him as a baby. He responded indirectly by turning to his mother to ask her for crackers. At moments like this Corey was still very difficult to "read." Did I cause a "play disruption" by offering to feed the elephant, or did my reference to "food" make him think of being fed himself and thus crackers? Moreover when he turned to his mother, he used a word instead of gesturing, "Op!" (Open), which in any case I thought should elicit a confirming response from us and thus treat the request at face value.

However, it was at times like this that not only did his mother and I read him differently, but we may have had different agendas, which must have confused him. In this instance Mrs. A tried to turn his request for crackers into a game, instead of simply giving him what he wanted, possibly because she thought to pursue "play" or possibly because she wanted to extinguish his insistence on eating in my office. He had indeed carried into our sessions the same passions for finding forbidden foods I had witnessed at home! I made an attempt to put this into words for both of them. I pointed out that perhaps my offering to feed a bottle to the elephant had made Corey think of us feeding him crackers. (Mrs. A and I had compromised by keeping a supply of special crackers that met Corey's dietary requirements.)

The elephant play showed developmental movement toward semi-symbolic play as well as clearer evidence of sequencing, or what we refer to as mini-modules of narrative and intentionality that show movement in the direction of pretend play. As we were coming to the end of the session, I announced "two more minutes," a warning I had recently introduced to help Corey transition out of the office. At that moment, he was sitting at the table and eating crackers. He seemed to reference my warning by initiating an "in and out" game. Then, upon getting ready to leave, Corey started to walk out with the elephant. Mrs. A, sounding harassed, began to negotiate taking it from him. Against my usual rules I thought it important he develop a transitional object and encouraged him to take it and also to bring it back.

SCHOOL VISIT

During the following week, I visited Corey's preschool. First I observed him through a one-way mirror. In a room with three teachers and several children, Corey was in his own world, unfocused in his affect. He made no eye-contact and avoided any instruction or social interaction. At the same time, he seemed very aware that the other children were doing things he wanted to do, and he tried to copy their actions without acknowledging them as people. His behavior was consistent with Baron-Cohen's observation that ASD children have an active sensory apparatus but cannot create the triangle of shared experience (Baron-Cohen, 1995).

When trying to copy his classmates' activities, he had little frustration-tolerance and his attempts were sometimes vague, subtle, and easily extinguished. After about 20 minutes, I entered the room and Corey approached me. Without looking at me he took my hand and led me to a dollhouse, where he put a father and boy together in a bed. Perhaps he was letting me know there was something he did know how to do. It was hard to tell whether he overall was avoidant out of performance anxiety, fear, or an inability to process his curiosity. It may have been all three.

DEVELOPMENTAL ADVANCES IN LANGUAGE (SIGN OF BEGINNING INDIVIDUATION) AND TOGETHERNESS

At the beginning of his third month of treatment I began to see the emergence of a sense of self and other in Corey's relationship to his mother, propelled by Corey's ability to pull away and be "different" from her. This was manifested in two ways, first by an increase in his ability to use language, particularly to have a word for "Mommy" (although he pronounced it like "Nanny"). Secondly, in the office, he initiated a game of "togetherness" that he played at home with his parents, in which they each held an arm and swung him. This seemed to be a compromise formation in that the three of them were implicitly separate, but dependent, people. Bringing this game into the office was also important in that it was one of the first references Corey made between us and his home life, a sign of increasing cognitive awareness in addition to his increasing ability to represent us in play. Similarly, after having made paper cut-outs of a "mommy car" and a "Corey car," Corey asked me to clip them together and carried them around with him.

Corey began to set the agenda of our sessions by initiating and then insisting upon repetition of segments of our play, books, and activities from one session to the next. He seemed to want to "review our repertoire," a shift that seemed multi-determined. For one it seemed to represent his increasing integration in the emotional/cognitive realm as he solidified representations of us as people. It also seemed to show progress from the physical game of "swinging togetherness" to a more semi-symbolic and truly representational, symbolic mode of play. Further, it may have also possibly comforted him that we could be "the same" every day in the face of Corey's exposure to changes taking place at home as his mother began to date. His once regularly scheduled visits with his father were also in flux, which led to visitations in his father's apartment instead of his father visiting him in his mother's apartment.

Most important to Corey in the "review" that began each session was reading several books to which he had become much attached. One constant was his need to find pictures of elephants, an interest his mother had introduced in our very first session. "Corey loves elephants," she had said. I had found that hard to believe at the time, given how impossible it was to read almost anything about what he liked in the way of toys or animals. Thus I read his current interest to suggest a measure of compliance. He had unconsciously internalized "choices" and "preferences" that stemmed from his mother's perceptions and needs. Another such preference was fascination with a panda family "sleeping" together, perhaps a representation derived from his dawning concerns about separation. Similarly he was averse to a picture in one of his favorite books of a 1950s-style mother holding her baby. I wondered if the representation was too jarring, as she looked so unlike his mother. Was his response perhaps a form of delayed stranger anxiety, emerging in the course of his shifting in the developmental process? I wondered too if this picture stirred conflict about individuating, emanating from his current concerns.

Concurrently Corey began to demonstrate developmental progress in other areas, showing fledgling interest in urination. At home, whenever his diaper was removed, he had begun peeing indiscriminately on the floors and rugs. When he started spilling cups of water in my office, I labeled this as "making pee-pee," noting (to myself) Mother's inappropriate laxity about Corey's messing at home and in the office compared to her hypervigilance about foodstuff. I began to work with Mrs. A. About not being afraid to set limits, including toilet-training.

In the middle of our third month, when Corey happened to be brought to a session by his father, he very clearly said "Sherkow" for the first time. I speculated he could do so because his mother was absent. Mr. A criticized Mrs. A for not allowing Corey to drink tap water and "eat so many crackers and raisins." He objected to her objections. Clearly understanding and identifying with his father's criticism, Corey yelled, "Jump on Mommy!"

SLEEP TRAINING AND TOILET-TRAINING PROGRESS

After a weeklong vacation, Corey showed evidence of another developmental leap. During the hiatus Corey had added to his vocabulary a clearer version of "Mommy" (still pronounced "Nanny") as well as a clearer "open," "up," "down," and "eat tummy," a replacement for "kiss elbow." Games that enacted separation themes expanded to include urinary, anal, and sleeping-alone themes, particularly by using raisins for "in-out play" of all kinds, including dumping them into the sink and toilet. In representational "sleep" play, he lay on my couch, which play I expanded by covering him, saying "Ah, Corey is sleeping!" Copying me with glee, Corey instructed his mother to lie down and "Sleep!" Agreeably she complied, and as I patted her hair, I said, "Mommy is sleeping!"

Corey grinned and climbed on the arm of the couch to stand over his mother. He looked like he was about to literally "Jump on Mommy." Experimenting with trying to turn this action into pretend play, I whispered to him, "Let's pretend: ready; set; go!" Corey giggled and stopped himself from jumping, enjoying the "pretend."

This play enabled Corey to move the game forward a step, introducing another element: "Mommy, wake up!" After many repetitions and turn-taking at being put to sleep and woken up, Corey elaborated this theme in a game of leaving us by going in and out of the office door, clearly linking spatial separation with the sleep-separation. Yet once again I observed that Mrs. A miscued his play by referring to it as "hide and seek," reflecting her struggle with his growing up, especially sleeping alone.

Corey followed this sequence by repeatedly dumping water into a toy toilet, seemingly confirming interest in urinary control. Moreover he followed this play with saying, "Taxi," now connecting bodily separations with traveling to and from my office. He proceeded to name the characters in one of his favorite books, showing me how "grown-up" he was becoming! My sense in these sessions was that Corey showed evidence of increasing individuation, internalizing commands to regulate himself. He showed both self-control and pleasure in being more mature, partially a consequence of his and his mother's therapy helping him feel safe in doing so. It was also interesting that Mrs. A's misunderstanding him did not disrupt his play, but rather he pursued his agenda.

THE REPRESENTATION OF THE DISAPPEARING MOMMY

In the next several weeks Corey expanded these themes, experimenting with his awareness of his bowel movements and the emerging anxiety about separating from both urine and stool. He continued to try to spill water whenever the opportunity presented itself and made frequent trips to the bathroom to deposit raisins or crackers. In the middle of playing "sleep," he hid his mother behind a pillow and wouldn't let her emerge. He then made me go to sleep without "wake-up." It became apparent that he, red-faced and inward gazing, was trying to move his bowels (in his diaper) right in front of us, a variation of the child who typically hides in a corner to move his bowels. I said, "Corey is trying to have a poop in front of us but doesn't want us to see him!" now understanding the earlier behavior of keeping *us* hidden.

Corey responded to my interpretation by the following fascinating sequence: he announced "Kitchen!" and grabbed a box of Pringles. He lined these precious, forbidden chips on the counter; he took the chips into the bathroom and dropped a chip down the toilet; and he put his finger in the toilet bowl, put a chip in the toilet bowl, and gingerly reached in to touch it. I imitated him, and he pushed the chip to the bottom of the bowl. Taking this cue, I flushed the toilet and said, "All gone, chip went bye-bye." Taking a handful of chips, he left the bathroom to hide the chips under the couch cushions, all the while avoiding looking at his mother. Seeing that he suddenly looked very unfocused and confused, I remarked, "Corey is making sure that mommy doesn't disappear!" He responded by saying, "Sing!" I thus sang, "Mommy's here, she didn't disappear!" to which he laughed, demanding numerous repetitions, after which he tried to push me out the door. From outside I sang, "Knock, and knock! Sherkow disappeared! Open the door!" as I went in and out of the office.

Soon I realized he was still pushing very hard to move his bowels and that I could represent his dual wishes to push me out of the room and his bowel movement out of his body by using bang-a-ball. I said "push, push" to the balls, but although he did push them down the chute, his affect was subdued. I wondered if, at this very moment, I was observing his turning inward as he concentrated on defecating.

Within these play themes about bodily and parent-child separation, Corey also showed more mastery of language. He rapidly added *Mickey Mouse*, *Donald Duck*, *empty*, *inside*, *cookie*, *water*, and *on/off* to his vocabulary. He showed more complex and subtle reactions, teasing me, and found ways to avoid or shut me out to express the negativity of the "terrible twos" by contrast to his earlier aversive behavior. In another correlate to the struggle one sees in the "anal" phase, Corey showed true ambivalence in trying to form responses to questions: he started to clap his hands to mean both "no" and "yes," seemingly not yet willing to learn those words. He also showed clear reactions that expressed his wishes, fears, or anxieties, such as putting his hands over his ears when his mother tried to sing familiar and favorite songs. While neither his mother nor I understood the meaning of this aversion, he let me invent a new song for us to use before the end of the hour: "Mommy isn't disappearing!"

SHUT-DARK

I knew that Corey struggled at home with falling asleep alone and staying in his bed all night. My supposition was that his difficulty processing bedtime, once a byproduct of his neurofunctional inability to comprehend the patterns involved in bedtime and boundaries, was now a byproduct of conflict. He was now "aware" of the difference between parts of his day: where he will sleep and with whom; who will let him into his/her bed; and his awareness of someone else perhaps being in his mother's bed. My guess was that he was conflicted about controlling and being controlled by his mother. He latched onto the phrase "Noises everywhere" (from *Good Night Moon*) as a signifier for these over-determined sleeping issues and arrangements.

By the end of the fourth month Corey had evolved in his play to symbolically represent his control over his parents and his orifices through more imaginative use of toys. In an important session, he was fascinated that he could erect a "barrier" to prevent cars and people from sliding down a ramp, and when he stopped them, he said "shut-dark" to signify holding them back, an apparent condensation of "holding poop back" and "being in the dark."

Near the end of the session he rolled the "mommy-baby" car down the couch and followed it with another, larger car. Reflecting on the stories Mrs. A had told me about tension between her and Mr. A in front of Corey, I asked Corey if the large car was the "Daddy car." He giggled and made the two cars crash into each other multiple times. After several minutes, however, he became tentative. He looked back toward mother, giving me the sense he might be hesitating to express aggression when it involved his father. He may even have hesitated to mention his father's name in front of his mother.

The next variation on the theme of exploring "shut-dark" was to play at opening and shutting doors of all kinds, to the play houses, the hospital, and the closet, to which I commented, labeling his actions, "You are opening the door to let the poopy balls through!" He used the phrase "shut-dark" every time we closed any door. After about a week of this play, Corey for the first time asked to "go poop" when outside his house.

However, Mrs. A became non-compliant to my request she refrain in our sessions from asking Corey if he wanted to use the potty, which had increasingly caused disruptions and negativity. He would become distracted and disorganized as soon as she brought it up. One kind of negativity took the form of his requesting chips but leaving them uneaten. I wondered if he was afraid of food prompting a reflex to defecate, which he seemed to resist in my office.

In another developmental push, Corey had developed a larger vocabulary but now demonstrated echolalia. He repeated speech sounds, partially enunciated words, and words he already had. I saw this as a component of his neurobiological processing deficiency, which perhaps was only becoming evident now he was rapidly trying to expand his language skills. Curiously Mrs. A treated his echolalic vocalizations as a game, encouraging them as though she were encouraging expanding his play. I shared with her my view she should inhibit his echolalia whenever possible and that we should attempt to understand his speech "no matter what," making meaning out of his sounds or repeated words even if we were incorrect. I explained that the act of making meaning in itself is helpful to him. I wondered if her "game-making," which seemed more like a regressive "joining" rather than creating communication and narrative, both demonstrated her difficulty understanding his symptoms and suggested she was resisting Corey's individuation.

DAWNING AWARENESS OF HIS GENITALIA, "OTHERNESS," AND MY MOMMY

In a session in the midst of our fifth month of treatment, Corey, now 30 months old, came into the office after having tried to make "Pee-pee on the potty" at home. He wanted to take off his diaper and demonstrate on my toilet, very pleased with himself. He was engrossed with putting "poopy balls" in a diaper and toy potty, and for the first time Corey joyfully shared with us an entire narrative about poop, as roughly follows: "Me not wanting to give up poop, and poopy balls go into diaper, and poopy balls go into the potty!"

A little later in the hour he became interested in my toy hospital and, for the first time, looked between the legs of a black rubber boy doll very intently for several seconds. When children do so, they typically are searching for genital information. Some minutes later, after playing with the bang-a-balls, putting them through doors and calling them "poopy-balls," Corey seemed to grab his genital area through his clothing and pull up, suggesting he might be feeling his penis or want to touch it. I said so, but Mrs. A contradicted me. It was the first indication that Mrs. A would not allow us to mention "penis." As far as she was concerned, he couldn't possibly be interested in his genitals, and I must be speaking from a Freudian perspective with which she did not agree. She openly derided me, going forward, whenever I came close to drawing attention to the clear evidence of Corey's genital interest.

The next week, his mother reported in front of Corey that he had shown a shift in his relationships with other children. For the first time during a play-date he seemed to understand his "friend" was a separate person who wanted to borrow Corey's elephant. Comprehending his mother's narrative, Corey struggled to put his newfound possessiveness into words. He turned to me and said, "This is *my* mommy."

Picking up dolls and a dollhouse, I enacted the scenario his mother had described and spoke his feelings for him. To this he associated new play behavior. He alternately rubbed or banged two dolls together, which I labeled "hugging" and "fighting." I sensed Corey's continuing preoccupation with whom he shared his mother, which likely mirrored his father's feelings. Although Mrs. A tried to keep her dating private, Mr. A had likely made his feelings known to Corey. He was very unhappy about the break-up.

Pursuing the themes of separation, autonomy, and self-regulation, I felt it was appropriate to address with both Corey and Mrs. A the overall issue of privacy. I strongly urged her to keep bathroom and bedroom doors shut and to keep Corey out of her bedroom altogether, and tolerate his whining or even his hysterics if necessary. Going forward, I began adding such scenarios to our play, enacting that both Corey and Mommy need their privacy.

Corey was brought to our next session by both parents, unplanned and unannounced to him, and he seemed very distracted and distressed, wearing a plastic smile. It seemed to me to be very confusing to him to have both parents present without warning, particularly in the context of their ongoing dissension and custody issues. Neither he nor I could understand their agenda, and I found myself thinking that Corey's plastic smile reflected the "phoniness" of this "togetherness." There was no possibility for Corey to engage in pretend play. There were "too many feelings" in the room, and too many people as well. Corey could not process their latent tension, and I was mystified as to where a potent feeling of "disapproval" was coming from and at whom it was directed. Not surprisingly, Corey demanded food, and after eating ravenously, threw chips all over my office rug. While Mrs. A sat passively, Mr. A told Corey to stop. This combination Corey apparently took as an invitation to test us, changing his facial expression into "teasing." He immediately dumped more chips!

Mrs. A interposed gleefully, "Now you are in for it!"

Following her "instruction," Corey stepped on toys and stomped on and crushed the chips, to which I announced, "Corey is angry! Corey is throwing things because he is angry!" After a few seconds' delay, Corey repeated this new word, "Angry!"

Mother's remark had signaled permission for Corey to express her anger at me. I delayed by proceeding simply to narrate the session's enactments. I recounted first my surprise at both parents coming—their wearing signs of disapproval, Corey's distractibility and anxiety, and then his anger and confusion about why his parents were both there (refraining from adding, "on the warpath"). In response to all this, Corey picked up small plastic figures representing his mother, his father, himself, and me and put "us" onto a spinning "rotator" on top of the toy garage, arranging and rearranging us into different family groupings: him, his mother, his father, and me; him only with father; him only with mother; and triangles that included me. This went on for at least five minutes, showing me he clearly understood the dilemma of them fighting over him in some way that also involved me.

Following his lead, Mrs. A wondered aloud if Corey was responding to a big fight his parents had had the previous night. Had Corey heard them in his sleep? I recounted my narrative of the session, adding this important detail and enacting his confusion and rage in reaction to their fighting. Moments later Corey grabbed an aerosol can of bath foam out of his mother's bags. For the second time in that hour, instead of limit-setting, Mrs. A declared, "Dr. Sherkow will have a good time with this!"

Paralyzed, I tried to intervene, but Corey raced to the bathroom and pressed the foam button directly into his mouth. Mrs. A laughed, which baffled me, while Mr. A expressed immediate concern about Corey swallowing foam. As both of them seemed, each in their own way, utterly passive, I attempted to clean Corey, but he escaped, rushed back into the bathroom, and again squirted foam into his mouth, which mother again ignored. Corey appeared to be begging his parents to apply rules and limit-setting to themselves. His power and freedom to act out must have been terribly anxiety-provoking, overwhelming, and had the potential to lead to self-injury.

I reserved my discussion with them about their anger, including their anger at me, until we met for our parent sessions. Unfortunately, I achieved no clarity other than their ongoing ambivalence, Mrs. A's extreme need to control Mr. A, and how these took a toll on Corey's ability to feel like he could "have both of them together," as he so clearly symbolized during the hour. Mrs. A's anger at me seemed a projection of her disappointment and inadequacy onto me, the idealized parent.

DEVELOPING A TRANSITIONAL OBJECT: A TEENAGE BOY DOLL

After Corey spent a weekend with his father, at age 31 months, Mr. A reportedly asked Mrs. A whether there was something wrong with their son's penis, because Mr. A had witnessed Corey playing with it all weekend. Like mother he seemed to see Corey as "asexual" or too infantile to be able to experience pleasure in exploring his genitals. Corey's play in my office was consistent with his interest in playing with his penis and exposed his anxiety about doing so, insofar as he became preoccupied with the concept of "broken."

Despite Mrs. A's denial, I had pointed out in our play how often Corey worried about toys or people being broken, toys falling apart, and furniture being wobbly. I had also shared with her that he had been engineering accidents with his body by treating furniture as "slippery." Having now heard of his father's denial as well, I wondered what effect it had on him for both parents to see him as being "gender neutral."

In a parallel development, Corey had fallen in love with a cartoon group of singers who had been made into 12-inch cloth dolls and who could be partly undressed. Corey reportedly slept with his "Anthony doll" now that his mother refused to let him sleep with her. Being able to accept an Anthony doll as a consistent transitional object, a substitute for his mother's snuggling with him, was an important development. Acquiring a transitional object, albeit belatedly for his actual age, was consistent with his developmental age, now in the midst of acquiring self-object differentiation (Winnicott, 1962).

Corey began to use his Anthony doll in the manner of neurotypical children, bringing Anthony everywhere he went, including to our sessions where Corey used him for the semi-symbolic play of putting Anthony through his own struggles, parenting him, and treating him like a friend. Once a transitional object was established, Corey was able to advance to independently getting himself ready for bed, brushing his hair and teeth, and taking his "Anthony" to sleep, separating from his mother now without protest.

After a two-week vacation, Corey returned with a new repertoire of ways to demonstrate anger at his mother. For some time he had been willing to defecate into a potty but now refused, demanding a diaper for that purpose, although he continued to use a potty for urinating on condition that he himself initiated it. If his mother requested that he go, he would have an accident rather than comply.

In place of his teasing games of jumping on mommy when distressed, Corey began hurting her by pulling her hair, or sticking his fingers into her mouth. When I tried to engage Mrs. A in conversation about this, she insisted Corey's show of negative emotion was subconscious but did not mean that he was angry! Consequently she was averse to my discussing his anger or its meaning with Corey, thus indirectly permitting him to continue to be angry and inflict pain. At the same time I saw he had begun to use the arms of my sofa couch as if he were standing on a windowsill, on the brink of falling through space. I speculated he was regressively expressing feeling cast aside and being made to disappear rather than be engaged with his mother in working through his normal, angry, and frustrated feelings. Her denial of his emotions likely made him feel obliterated while also diminishing my role as a helping object. This froze me out from making interpretations.

BACKLASH BY CUTTING BACK SESSIONS

It became apparent that Mr. A was successfully individuating from Mrs. A, and, in the process, Corey was becoming more attached and comfortable with him. From Mrs. A's point of view I was to blame, and in fact I was vulnerable to being demoted from Corey's team. Without consulting me, Mrs. A gave away three of our weekly hours to other activities and types of therapy, expecting that I would be able to accommodate her. Left to scramble for new times to see Corey, so as not to victimize him, our frequency was reduced to plus or minus two sessions for most of the month in which Corey was beginning a new pre-school. Corey protested, apparently, after about two weeks of his new schedule. Mrs. A called and told me that Corey had mentioned how much he loved his sessions with me. Because, she had now realized, he had made such significant progress during our work together she wanted me to reinstate our former schedule.

I experienced in Mrs. A's transference to me that she longed to be beloved by a maternal figure whom she had experienced as withholding and punitive and who did not validate her feelings of either love or hate. As a result she was prone to forming rigid, fragile rationalizations and intellectualizations to defend against disappointment, with sadistic urges asserting themselves "out of the blue." These outbursts had the same random and disruptive quality I had seen in Corey when he was confronted with his own angry and rejecting feelings.

THE BEGINNING OF NARRATIVE PLAY

Corey soon took another developmental leap in his language ability at 32 months. He began to create narratives, using full sentences, as we engaged in pretend play. He no longer showed echolalia in his speech patterns. For example, when he came to a session while his mother was in the hospital following surgery for a broken wrist, he pulled out the toy hospital, played at putting a mother into a bed, and asked for help in putting a Band-Aid on her. (He had not used the hospital for some time.) He segued from this scenario to taking down the dollhouse, with which he played "Go in?" and "Don't go in, it's dark and scary!"

Father, who had brought him, interjected, "Over the weekend Corey stood up and pooped in the bathtub!" I responded by saying to them this must have been Corey's way of showing he wanted to hang onto his poop, not wanting to lose anything by flushing something important down the toilet, just as he was afraid of losing Mommy, hurt, in the hospital. To this Corey grabbed his crotch several times and picked up several small, hard dolls. He tried to put these into his pants. I labeled this action and asked Mr. A whether Corey had been touching his penis when in Dad's presence. "Yes, in the sauna," he said. "I am trying to show him how to pee standing up." I remarked this was helpful for Corey, and we played at making a boy doll stand and pee on a potty.

Further progress in Corey's individuation in the presence of his father was evidenced in our next session when Corey picked up a zoo book and positioned a male rubber doll to stand on the pages of the book. He said to the doll as a parent might to a child, "Look, this is a tiger. Look, this is a giraffe. Look, the giraffes are eating hay… behind the fence." I understood him reflecting what his father had said: the boy standing up to urinate, able to look at and show off his genitals from the perspective of urinating in a toilet. He identified with his father's pride in him and his progress. In addition he spent some time in each session trying to make three figures hold hands or hug with a driven, anxious quality; most likely responding to the mixture of hugging, representing his father's allying himself with me around Corey's successes, and anxiety at being disloyal to his mother.

TALKING IN WHOLE SENTENCES AND TELLING ME WHAT HE WANTS

Corey had advanced in his play to the point where he could operate the toy garage elevator on his own, a milestone. He then narrated through play with the dollhouse a story of his grandpa going to the hospital: the doctor was fixing him, and Daddy was going on an airplane. We had a conversation about his missing his father when he was away on a business trip.

When, soon after, both parents came to a session, Corey became very excited, putting several naked dolls on his stomach. Then he asked his parents to sit on the floor with him and sent me out of the room, closing the door behind me! I interpreted that he loved having Mommy and Daddy alone with him. A little later he sought a box of animals and put three horses together excitedly. Just then Mrs. A stood to go the bathroom and Corey just howled. I said he was very unhappy that mother disrupted our play just when he was going to put the three horses together and that he really loved having Mommy and Daddy together and was angry at the interruption.

The next day Corey cried in the hallway, refusing to come into the office. I interpreted he had been upset the day before when his play with Mommy and Daddy alone was disrupted and he was letting me know how he felt. Mrs. A acted like I was nuts, but Corey was far more engaged during the rest of the session, doing his ABCs and playing with the musical instruments. As I had intervened earlier in the week, telling Mrs. A she cannot be on the phone during our sessions, she played with us. Joyfully he initiated reciprocal play with the musical instruments.

Another example of his developmental leap in language and play skills was his newfound ability to discuss his schedule not by rote but by understanding the concepts of "before and "after," time of day, and the sequence of days in the week. This allowed him to describe the narrative of his weekend. He understood he had a "vacation house" and could talk about bringing his dog to visit his grandfather's house. However, his speech patterns were not yet normalized in total. There was still some residual echolalia, not always easy to pinpoint as connected to anxiety or conflict. Now Corey was also consistently clear about what he wanted to eat and what he wanted to play, and he increasingly used playthings to symbolize. For example, in addition to the frequent "putting poopy balls in the diaper," he hid the balls under the couch and said, "They are going on vacation!" His repertoire of doll play also expanded: he now used rubber figure dolls to represent his grandparents.

Corey could now express his anger directly at me, for example, when I denied him crackers. He also regularly teased me about whether he could touch the "grown-up" scissors. "Not safe," he would say, mirroring my earlier confrontation. His mother remarked that, in fact, he had told his speech therapist that "Sherkow says scissors aren't safe" in a clear example of the necessary developmental marker (Baron-Cohen, 1995) of triangulation of joint attention. Similarly, he presently struggled with the concept of me/mine, both with reference to himself and to me and my office.

Socially, Corey had made significant progress in having play dates and interacting with other children at his playgroup. His behavior in less structured environments, such as a playground, continued to be mixed. He was increasingly prone to hugging strange children, whom he might later push. Mrs. A had begun to apply to nursery schools without discussing this directly with Corey, who must have understood that "something is happening." Yet she refused to let me talk to him about the transition as though it didn't exist if we didn't call attention to it, which frustrated my attempts to help Corey manage transitions and learn to anticipate in order to organize himself and foster self-regulation.

Upon their return from a weeklong vacation, Corey's play showed another developmental leap: he consistently played with toys in making mini-modules that demonstrated his progression to labeling, "sorting," "categorizing," and sequencing, consistent with typical 24-month-old toddler behavior. He was still exquisitely sensitive to his mother's comments, and she consistently miscued his behavior. For instance, as he labeled and sorted toy fruit, she loudly remarked that she had told his play-group director how well he plays with me, comparing herself negatively.

Corey reacted by throwing the fruit and silverware over the back of the play kitchen. While I tried to help him handle the conflict she presented, which I believed led him to anxiously "throw" the toys, Mrs. A laughed and said he was mimicking "throwing fish to the sharks," something they had just done on their vacation. Such indirect encouragement of Corey's unacceptable behavior continued to confuse us both.

AWARENESS OF SEQUENCES: TIME, SCHEDULES, AND INTERNALIZATION

As Corey and I approached the end of that week, he picked up a pen, marched over to my appointment book, and pointed out, accurately, which days he was coming during the upcoming week. "No Sherkow. No Sherkow. Yes Sherkow. Yes Sherkow."

For the first time he used the word "together." He had advanced to talking in complete sentences, and could describe the past, talk about the future, and express his wishes. Corey's play also increasingly represented his experiences. For example, he used little dolls to narrate going to the park, telling me they were swinging on the "big-boy" swing, instead of the baby swing. Another time he hid a doll under my couch and said, "I am sending the baby on vacation!" Because our new schedule included a day when he ate lunch in my office, he brought a "picnic" once a week and we ate together on the office carpet.

One such lunchtime, he arrived carrying his "picnic lunch" but immediately grabbed and happily ate my chicken, ignoring his own food. While we ate he sorted the musical instruments, playing orchestra with me. He had developed a fascination with their various sounds, and we regularly made up songs to express our feelings. He asked me to play a CD to which we had danced on earlier occasions, looking for the track of a song I particularly liked. "Ah," I said, "you not only enjoyed eating my chicken, but you also want to play my favorite song!"

Giggling like crazy, he said, "It's my favorite song is Sherkow's song! [*sic*]" Following this he anxiously announced, "Jump on Mommy!"

Understanding his dilemma, I said, "You are worried about saying that your favorite song was 'Sherkow's song.' You want to make sure that Mommy knows you love her best!" He then hugged me, still clinging to me as he jumped over a table into her lap. As they were leaving, he grabbed my chicken bone and demanded to take it home! When I learned he had a bowel movement on the adult toilet at his father's house that evening, I understood that milestone as confirmation of the work he had done to develop a stable sense of self in the face of "loaded" transitions.

DRAWING TO EXPRESS EMOTIONS

With his advancement in cognitive skills and processing information, Corey by 33 months became able to learn his letters, to sit through reading books cover-to-cover, and to allow me to use drawings to express his experiences. For example, as he was now applying to schools, each new interview threw him into a state of confusion. He became clingy during transitions to his scheduled activities, especially play-group, and suddenly became phobic of one of his helpers when he accidently saw her out of context on the sidewalk. I drew stick figures for him, naming each of them as a child in his group in the hope of identifying them in representations that would help him to process "old friends" and "new friends," current teachers and prospective teachers.

As we labeled the "old friends," he pointed to two of them as "Corey."

Puzzled at first, I thought and then said, "Oh, I see, there are a happy Corey and a sad Corey." Delighted, he proceeded to let me help him make stick figures for many more upsetting emotions: angry Corey, worried Corey, and so forth. This became a technique we then could usefully and magically apply to many people and situations going forward. Not only would he want me to draw them, but he would then share making faces and trying on different expressions.

ACHIEVING "THEORY OF MIND": THE DEVELOPMENT OF EPISTEMIC MECHANISMS

By 34 months, Corey would more frequently be dropped off and attend his sessions alone. He was increasingly able to put his struggle with his mother's beliefs and attitudes into his play and now able to turn his oppositional behavior into a game, a surprising and sudden leap into abstraction which showed he understood he was being intentionally oppositional in school, for example, when he would be chronically chastised for trying to eat forbidden Play-Doh.

In Baron-Cohen's terms, through Corey's frequent attempts to fool me in his play, we saw the beginning of epistemic mechanisms: pretending, thinking, guessing, deceiving, and thus joking (Baron-Cohen, 1995). In one scenario, he would set up two dollhouses, one belonging to Mom and one to Dad. He would then deceive me about where he was going to sleep, "torturing" me in the role of one parent or the other, by making me worried that he was lost, suspicious, or angry at me for some misdeed, particularly enacting jealousy over where he preferred visitation. On an occasion when he had been dropped off by his mother, he played that his father was taking him on a special vacation; I knew the vacation father had planned was vetoed by his mother. When she arrived to pick him up, he told her point blank that he wanted to go on vacation with Daddy. She immediately turned on me for having "put this idea in his head!" It was easy to read on Corey's face that he was thrilled that I was getting the rap for his having expressed his wishes!

It was not surprising then that soon after that hour Corey announced "I am happy at Sherkow's!" He was also learning how to anticipate the thoughts and feelings of others, including his Mother, by not only anticipating his mother's reaction to his requests but also anticipating her bad moods by preemptively asking her for a kiss, which required processing multiple representations of self and other. He was able to express feeling scared of his mother and worried about being punished for being naughty, while at the same time he loved to play at thwarting her during those sessions in which we met without her.

For example, he took out the musical instruments, and, pretending he was playing a violin, while I played a xylophone, we marched around our picnic circle, paper plates and all, while he elaborately described his intent to eat everything his mother denied him. "I'll eat gluten and I'll eat dairy and I'll eat ice cream, chocolate, candy." The two of us laughed hysterically like incredibly naughty children about to be caught stealing cookies out of the jar. He could also talk openly about feeling scared of her because of something naughty he has done or wants to do, expressing his anxiety and expectation of being punished.

DISCUSSION

During the course of the next year, Corey continued to develop both receptive and expressive language skills, using multisyllabic words, and could fully narrate his past and present experiences. He evolved to the point that he showed an excellent memory, frequently referring to experiences he'd had months past, contextualizing them accurately and meaningfully in the present. The latter included his awareness of his and other's affective states and his awareness of his bodily functions.

When his parents began a consolidated effort to set guidelines for Corey's good and bad behavior, he very quickly made it clear that he understood the transition toward self-regulation and discipline and showed remarkable ability to identify and internalize what was being asked of him, understanding and obeying rules.

Corey continued to be a loving, demonstrative child, who readily engaged his family and therapists. He also readily engaged children and adults that were well known to him, although he still struggled to make social contact with children when in a group, despite being sometimes almost desperate to do so. While once he would have approached children he wanted to know by inappropriately hugging them, or "being in their face," he now tended to be passive and observant. He showed much less difficulty with impulse control, would no longer grab, hit, or spill under duress, and was not prone to temper tantrums unless extremely stressed. I observed him, in his new school, sitting quietly in an auditorium and attending to music class and a dramatic production, not overstimulated as he once would have been by "unknown" situations or people. He continued to be free of any idiosyncratic, perseverative, or stereotypic behaviors.

I hope this case makes clear the importance of working with the dyad. While Mrs. A at times did not engage with me around the behavioral modeling cues offered by this kind of treatment, that is, modeling affective interactions between analyst and child, she seemed able to internalize my work sufficiently to allow Corey space for separation and development, including his ultimate ability to form an intimate relationship with his father.

Corey shows an example of how neurofunctional impairment might impede acquisition of representations necessary to establish boundaries and awareness of cause and effect. In Corey's case, his mother's style and need to be more competent than the idealized analyst compounded his problem, prolonging the conflict in his relationship to an ambivalently held object. Corey needed to achieve enough individuation to modulate his loving and hostile feelings toward his mother, an integration essential for transitioning to wanting her as his oedipal, not oral, object.

SOME OBSERVATIONS ABOUT AGGRESSION AND ITS ROLE IN MENTALIZING THE OTHER

I found it significant that language emerged during several week-long interludes between sessions, suggesting that these separations played a role in organizing a cognitive/emotional representation of me, as a byproduct of intense feelings of aggression toward me, that led to a developmental leap and consolidation of progress. This has been described in the literature wherein patients become "lucid" and lose their symptoms during a bout of angry feelings (Evered, 2011).

I wonder about the mechanism of action in a clinical setting, since it seemed to be the case in my work with Corey. I speculate that identifying intense feelings of aggression and connecting those feelings to an object, in this case me, could be an organizer of neuronal processes that allow emotion to connect to pathways of representing feelings and ideas, freeing up the ability to form interpersonal connections. I wonder if the implicit sense of "absence" during an interruption plays a role in ego development by virtue of an increased cathexis of the negative feelings, which, when identified in the analytic setting, can be represented in words on the way to promoting symbolization. Does a reunion diminish anxiety arising out of conflict, that being the mechanism of action? Corey's reactions bring to mind our hypothesis outlined in the introduction to the volume: does a neuronal deficit interfere with the process of categorizing patterns, from integrating his "like" experiences? Or, alternatively, does anger increase the ability to "read" meaning, and hence facilitate integration? In either case, the positive neurofunctional outcome could be seen as a new-found ability to make meaningful assessments and integrations of previously disconnected experiences into schema that serve to increase the functional capacity for symbolic development.

Chapter Four

Ethan

PRELUDE

Ethan's parents worried throughout Ethan's second year whether their son might be "on the spectrum." When during an extensive consultation the interviewers apprised that Ethan likely met the criteria of ASD, his parents reacted with such alarm that Ethan became immediately more gaze averse, avoidant, and non-responsive than he had been prior to the consultation.

From age 1 to 2 years, Ethan's parents had found him to be a ubiquitously cheerful, seemingly social toddler who had acquired a precocious degree of vocabulary and a facility with numbers and letters that was deceptively reassuring. However, Ethan's inability to use language skills to communicate or respond to them worried his parents. In addition, although he could easily transition from one caregiver to another, and had shown no "separation" reactions, he erupted readily into temper tantrums. His sociability with adults contrasted with an apparent lag in interpersonal skills with other children, showing no interest in "parallel play." Instead, he was obsessed with playing CDs, and was dependent on a stack of CDs and DVDs for purposes that were unclear. Thus, Ethan was most noticeably uneven in the areas of his object-relations and the acquisition of cognitive, language, and symbolic processing skills preliminary to developing play and communication ability.

Alongside the category of "Autism Spectrum Disorder," we find in our practices another spectrum of "uneven development" where the children do not meet the criteria for a formal diagnosis and whose prognosis without intervention is unknowable. Although many children mature at different rates in acquiring competencies, some show sharper lags in one area in contrast to precocious maturation in another, which often raises a red flag for parents and pediatricians. Developmental unevenness can be very confounding for concerned parents who find it difficult to "read" their child, often impacting their ability to trust their parental instincts and manage expectations. As with a child with ASD, these children are typically confused, vulnerable, and potentially even averse to their parents' reaction to gaps in competencies, gaps of which they may or may not be implicitly aware. The gaps can act like "symptoms," affecting one's sense of "self," and can create insecurity and chronic anxiety in a mother's sense of attachment to her child and so affect the development of basic trust in both parent and child.

Ethan was such a toddler. His compliance and "adorable" demeanor masked his inability to cope with any negative feelings or experiences, which so threatened his equilibrium that he was thrown by aggression (his own or his parents') into an overwhelming state of distress manifest by intense, unremitting temper tantrums. He used language that appeared to be more like lingual fixations, devoid of meaning, which biased communication.

Developmental unevenness is puzzling, leaving the clinician to speculate whether, over time, the more classic triad of ASD will appear. Functionally the state of unevenness may worsen in the face of faltering parental expectations. When Ethan's parents began to "see" their son as "defective," already feeling defeated, they retreated from asking him to master a toddler's developmental tasks: toilet-training, tolerating frustration, delaying gratification, and evolving both reciprocal and pretend play.

Working with Ethan provided a glimpse into the processes of internalization and joint attention, which played a prominent role in his treatment. At the height of his working toward differentiating emotions, it appeared that I was watching Ethan in the process of internalizing his experience of me, a process that Klin describes as imbuing an action with meaning, as a result of the responses of the other (Klin, 2007). Ethan made meaning in his interactions with me by watching me react to him, then copying me, in the context of expressing intense emotion. This work of trans-representational interaction felt to me like an opportunity to see in action how "taking in" and "registering" representations of the other might be more than a hypothetical process.

THE EVALUATION

Ethan was brought to see me at age 28 months to reevaluate the prior diagnosis of presumptive ASD. He was the second of 2 children in an intact family; his father maintained a moderately busy schedule, and his mother had retired from working when their first child, a daughter 4 years older than Ethan, was born. There had been no complications during pregnancy, birth, or during the first 12 months of Ethan's life, nor was there any family history of ASD. When he was about 12 to 14 months, his parents became concerned that

Ethan did not seem to be as responsive as they expected, gradually showed less interest in them, did not respond to his name, and seemed to show diminished use of language to express his needs. By about 2 years of age, what seemed like a "speech delay" appeared more serious, and his pediatrician agreed Ethan needed to consult with a language specialist. At this point, he was largely blocking his parents' requests and commands. He answered "no" only sometimes and indicated "yes" by mimicking the question several times.

Through initiating speech and language therapy, Ethan continued to develop words and an extensive vocabulary. Although he showed some improvement in responding to his name, he became hyperfocused on activities that interested him, like putting DVDs and CDs in and out of machines. He became obsessed with his mother's credit cards but "tuned the rest of the world out." He showed himself to be "intellectually advanced," had learned letters, numbers, colors, and shapes with ease, and reportedly was fantastic at puzzles. Yet he avoided other children. He played in the same room as his older sister without really interacting with her. He ignored her bids to join her in play. She was very sweet to him, defended him, and treated him like a pet. Ethan's parents harbored concerns regarding Ethan's social function, communicative language, and the presence of these obsessive and repetitive interests.

At 25 months, Ethan had been brought for a diagnostic evaluation at a major medical center. Ethan was present for the entire 2-hour evaluation and history-taking, overhearing everything that was said. He also must have observed his parents' reaction when the evaluator shared her hypothesis that Ethan fell just short of the criteria for autism. Ethan's parents left the evaluation "hysterical," and similarly, for the next two weeks, Ethan became utterly unresponsive to them, having tantrums and refusing to be soothed, leading to the referral to me.

Ethan's history revealed that his behavior at home was loving, and that he was typically a "giggly" happy boy who readily found humor in daily situations and on TV or videos. He could be put to bed easily and slept well, having never shown the sleep disruption or separation anxiety common in the second year. Ethan had little sense of his body, his body parts, his elimination, or of dressing or undressing himself, and resisted any prodding toward toilet training. He would finger feed himself but was a very picky eater. His mother had to hide meat and vegetables in his rigatoni in order to feed him something other than starch. To date, Ethan had shown no genital interest, either in touching his penis, referring to genitalia, responding to the genital differences he was exposed to with his sister and mother, nor shown any evidence that he differentiated between boys and girls.

Ethan's parents were very psychologically minded, and understood that he had already "learned" to "manage" his mother in particular by either demanding CDs or her credit cards, so that she bowed to his wishes rather than "fight" what seemed to her like a losing battle. If she resisted handing them over, or allowed even the slightest frustration in her voice at submitting to him, he became hysterical. The tantrums included hitting, biting, and pulling his mother's long hair.

Both parents were disturbed by Ethan's preoccupation with repetitive concrete tasks, mainly but not limited to putting CDs and DVDs into players, listening to them for a few minutes, and then taking them out, or sometimes only moving them in and out. Ethan showed a brilliant understanding of classical music and was able to distinguish a bar of Beethoven from Mozart. The metaphors of "rigid," "plastic," and "inflexible," as they applied to both Ethan and his CDs and credit cards, were not lost on his parents.

MEETING ETHAN

I met with Ethan for several evaluation sessions in the presence of his mother. As is my mode, I sat on the floor in the middle of a playroom, which is separated by a small waiting room from my "adult analytic" office. Ethan's mother sat alongside and we watched Ethan, and I watched both of them, engaging Ethan when appropriate, but not imposing any expectations on either of them. At first blush, one would take Ethan for being an utterly cheerful and charismatic little boy, but I quickly noticed the shallowness of his affect and how it obscured the fact that he did not actually make eye contact but blithely talked away in his little sing-song manner. I also noticed he walked on his toes, used my toys gingerly, and although he looked around at the toys, exploring boxes and shelves, he did not "play" with any one item, handling a toy telephone and a toy garage briefly, but showing no imaginative or narrative play. Ethan was very small for his age and was typically dressed like a little man, in clothes that seemed too binding and formal for a 2-year-old. He moved and climbed easily but could not jump.

I immediately also saw what his parents had described: not asking for help in having his needs met and instead seeking what he wanted on his own, even if he became frustrated in doing so. He could not spontaneously say, "I want X" off of the shelf, nor did he respond to social cueing, such as "waving bye-bye," saying "hi," or initiating hugs and kisses. I found Ethan as symptomatic as had been described with respect to his ability to directly relate, nor did he show any inclination to imitate my or his mother's actions. When pressed by his mother for an answer, he repeated sentences with no indication of meaning, and "yes" and "no" were absent from his vocabulary. Other than demanding CDs and his mother's credit cards, his communications were limited to labeling what he saw in the office in a high-pitched, inflexible cadence. He clearly grasped adult conversation and language concepts, both expressively and receptively. He displayed advanced fine motor but immature gross motor skills.

I found his parents' description of Ethan's sociability deceptive. In my office, his affect appeared two-dimensional, with little evidence of modulation between pleasure and distress. He navigated from one to the other using sing-song speech. I also observed that he was a "thumb sucker," readily turning to his thumb, and his mother's hair, for comfort.

Ethan's parents accepted my recommendation for dyadic therapy for Ethan and his mother on a four-times-per-week basis, with additional weekly sessions with his parents, and the addition of occupational therapy to his regimen of psychologically informed language therapy to work on his representational and affective use of language. He was already enrolled in a half-day nursery program in a very undemanding and nurturing setting.

BEGINNING THERAPY

During the first few weeks of our work, I became better acquainted with Ethan's affect and degree of relatedness to his mother. His demeanor was invariably "cheery and lovable," as his parents had described, unless he became frustrated, in which case he could turn immediately into a tantrum mode. He talked "at" or "around" us, which, along with his significant gaze aversion, made him seem more robotic than connected. I also saw, as had been reported, little modulation in the pitch of his voice, his movements, his mood, or his neediness. Although he had been described as attached and loving, there was little spontaneity in the hours. He paid little attention to either his mother or me during the first few days, and he behaved more or less like an inspector examining the scene. I tried to join him, where possible, but as he showed so little affect, it was hard to see where I could approach him in a meaningful way.

During the second week, Ethan approached me without making eye contact, wearing a mischievous grin. He brought some toys out of a bin and sat himself and the toys next to me on the floor. While he was not exactly "playing" with *me*, through his body language he seemed to be making a connection while subtly ignoring his mother. Over the next weeks, I watched Ethan develop an attachment to my office without my being able to discern what he was feeling. I could imagine that it was comfortable for him to come to a calm, non-demanding environment, and that the routine and the setting might be more meaningful to him than the quality of a relationship.

Generally, from the moment he entered the playroom, Ethan's facial expressions continued to be fairly rigid and his affect neutral to positive, seemingly "happy." His play with my toys had a rote quality: he would pick up the doctor's kit and pretend to examine me or his mother, giving us shots, or would ask to set up a train and watch it move along the tracks. He might pick up Fisher Price and other doll figures, which he would label indiscriminately with regard to gender.

Ethan seemed to take genuine pleasure only when pretending to talk on his mother's cell phone to his father or grandparent. By contrast, when his mother prodded him to "tell Dr. Sherkow" how he spent his day, or to describe their plans, Ethan would respond by stiffly echoing her questions, in a singsong intonation, keeping his back to us. Before long, I could see glimmers of performance anxiety emerging.

Most vividly, Ethan carried a stack of CDs and/or DVDs wherever he went—in his stroller, backpack, or his mother's bag. In coming into my office, he left them in his stroller in the waiting room. The door open, he would repeatedly interrupt himself in our "play" (which was hardly representational or pretend play) to check on them or ask his mother for reassurance they were still there. I wondered to what extent his discs were his "pals," his "transitional objects," or whether he had even arrived at that level of development in his object-relations. Clearly he used them to bridge transitions from one place to another, acting as if they were the only safe and sure element he could count on. In addition, his fixation with credit cards seemed to substitute for, or be a representation of, their relationship and an instrument he could use instead of words to control and punish his mother. Gradually, I saw more of his maladaptive, perseverative use of discs and credit cards. When very distressed he would hit, bite, or pull her hair. Otherwise, he seemed to have found a way to self-regulate by displacing his aggression onto a concrete object.

From parent sessions, I formed a clearer picture of the use and purpose of Ethan's perseverative use of CDs and credit cards. For example, instead of expressing feelings about leaving the house, traveling, or communicating his needs, he would insist on (and sometimes scream) for his mother's credit card to pay for their frequent taxi rides, allowing him to be in control of their travel by virtue of the rigid and unpredictable ways he would demand to have or use the credit card, as if paying for the taxi, controlling the transition into and out of the building or the cab, substituted for controlling his potential loss of his mother once he left the house. We began to see the pattern: all transitions out of the house were managed by the use of a credit card interaction; in the house, all transitions were managed by putting CDs and DVDs in and out of cases. Being brilliant about music and able to identify letters, Ethan recognized CDs by their covers, could name the composer, as well as recognize the music on each track, but could not seem to recognize patterns in his routine that would give him what he needed. My sense was that these pieces of plastic represented an inflexible substitute for more complex and meaningful interactions with his parents.

VISITING SCHOOL

I had the opportunity to observe Ethan in school behind a one-way mirror, where I saw him similarly manage transitions and separations through rigid and concrete behaviors. Upon entering the classroom, for the better part of the first semester, Ethan had accommodated to the transition to his classroom by slowly making the rounds of the pictures of each child pinned along the perimeter. In a sing-song intonation, he would recite the names of the children, their birthdays, their weekly tasks, and any other materials pinned to the pictures. He then would walk about the room to watch the children at their stations, and seemed particularly interested in watching them sing during "circle time," but he kept himself at a physical distance, and neither spoke to nor joined the other children in their activities.

PROCESSING BEING "STUCK"

I now had a grasp of the way Ethan's "unevenness" expressed itself, especially in relation to transitions. I watched him manage the obvious frightened feelings his mother displayed in our sessions, which to him was likely a form of overstimulation. It seemed possible that, in warding off one kind of overstimulation, he ultimately warded off all stimulation, and thus, biologically driven to take control, and exert his agency, he became stuck on CDs and credit cards. A more neurobiologically impaired ASD child might have taken to twirling or echolalia.

I began to wonder if Ethan also perceived his mother as "fixed" and "stuck." He certainly behaved as though he were impervious to the variety in her moods, affects, and expectations of him. I wondered if the modulations that I saw on a daily basis were functionally blocked and, if they registered to him at all, seemed just as arbitrary to Ethan. Ethan unquestionably could tell people apart. Baron-Cohen and others describe ASD children as retaining this facility even when they cannot attribute qualitative states to others, that is, are "mindblind." (Baron-Cohen, 2005; Klin & Jones, 2007)

I tried to find ways to point to, and label, any evidence of Ethan differentiating states of mind, moods, and interactions in our play. Ethan finally presented me with an opportunity when he began playing with my toy instruments. As he handed each of us an instrument, I began singing to the tune of Frère Jacques, "We make music, we make music, Dr. S and Mommy and Ethan, yes we do. Dr. S has the drum, and Ethan has the maracas, and Mommy has the flute!" At first Mrs. E and I sang while Ethan banged the drum, blew on the whistle, or shook the maracas, but after a number of sessions, Ethan began to sing along.

about missing me, and while leaning on me, also dictated a letter to his mother, who was sitting a few feet away, "Dear Mommy, when you go bye-bye I miss you, Love, E." It seemed at this moment he made a significant, positive therapeutic shift in being able to use his relationship with me to directly address his feelings about separating from his mother.

In the ensuing weeks, Ethan's most significant progress was recorded in these dictations. In December, as we were a week away from a two-week interruption for the Christmas holiday, Ethan, now 31 months, scribbled in red and black, "Dear Dr. Sherkow, I miss you when we stop." Turning over the page, he told me to write on the back, "I will be here on Friday!" He then had me start yet another letter, "Dear Dr. Sherkow, are you. . . ." but ran out of room without finishing his thought, seeming to express his anxiety about losing me. Perhaps he was also showing, in his concrete inability to frame his thoughts, his inability to see me as a separate person who was going to do something not only apart but also different from him. I saw this as an illustration of Ethan's struggle to form a "Theory of Mind," as if he were developing the ability to form a mental representation of me doing something outside his purview.

The following day, four days from the vacation, Ethan dictated, "Dear daddy, I miss you when you work." He added blue to his usual red and black scribble. Was that meaningful? Was be expanding his repertoire? Taking chances? How does one know when one is seeing the incremental steps in developing complexity?

PUTTING HIS ANGER AT MOMMY INTO WORDS

The next day, after playing a considerable amount of time with the Fisher Price dolls, including the "angry boy" figure, Ethan dictated, "Dear Dr. Sherkow, I am mad at Mommy," and again he scribbled in red, blue, and black. I said, "Yes, you feel angry at Mommy just like the 'angry boy' you were playing with before." I drew a facsimile of the "angry boy" figure. Leaning on me, he dictated, "Dear Dr. Sherkow, I am angry boy." It remained to be seen how much his anger would continue to be as denied, isolated, or dissociated!

A day later, the penultimate day before the holiday, Ethan scribbled and dictated, "Dear Dr. Sherkow, I make poo poo in my diaper," in a very obvious expansion in his communications to his mother! This was his first reference to his bowels, his fear of toilet-training, and his own body, and it seemed to reflect his anal concerns in relation to his anger at the upcoming separation. A bit later he challenged me by asking to use *adult* scissors to make cuts in the pad of paper. When I wouldn't let him do so, saying it wasn't safe, he became hysterical. Although he could barely be calmed enough to listen, I nevertheless wrote for him, “Dear Dr. Sherkow, I want the black scissors but Dr. Sherkow says no. I am going to see you tomorrow.” I understood his request for scissors as a displacement onto something concretely “unacceptable”—his unacceptable feelings toward me for letting him go on vacation.

In this vignette, one sees Ethan struggle with “new” awareness of feeling states but not yet be able to articulate his feelings in an age-appropriate way. The process of the fight over the scissors signified his wrestling with his worry about our separation, and the content of the fight (the grown-up scissors) signified his conflict about becoming a big boy. Practicing cutting the paper was a new developmental step, but fighting to tell us he wanted to be more grown-up (enough to use adult scissors) was expressed in an infantile tantrum instead of with words.

REPRESENTING HIMSELF AS SEPARATE

Upon Ethan’s return we saw multiple derivatives of his ambivalence about seeing himself as a person, as well as a separate person, as though he was integrating his newfound sense of self, from the neurobiological perspective, with his newfound sense of self from the object-relations perspective. While the first seemed to be welcome, the second was terrifying to him. In our first session after the break, Ethan, for the first time, scribbled while dictating, “Dear Dr. Sherkow, I do not like to be told what to do. I do it my way. I miss you.” This seemed to indicate his being able to now represent himself as a person who has agency. He could use the first person pronoun, describe himself both passively and actively, owning his wish to be in control. He also implicitly seemed to understand that asserting himself would precipitate a loss of his mother or me. The progress here was remarkable, in that he could now dictate the terms of separation and loss in words, compared to his feeling compelled to action in demanding scissors during the earlier struggle to protect against losing me.

Not surprisingly, the emerging development of a sense of separateness included “knowing” about, and thus “separating from” his body products, which he experienced with the same mixture of excitement and duress he had exhibited in mastering separation by insisting on the “grown-up” scissors. I received a telephone message from Mrs. E, who said, “This morning Ethan refused to let his me change his diaper. He was screaming, ‘No change my poopy!’ When I removed the dirty diaper, it took two of us to put on a clean one. Ethan screamed that he wanted to be changed back to the dirty diaper. My husband and I told him, ‘We understand that you are scared and angry.’ I finally just took the clean diaper off, and he immediately checked to make sure his penis was still there! This confirms our hypothesis, and adds weight to our guess that the renewed biting is connected to the fear of losing his precious genital in addition to his precious mommy and his precious poops . . . love it."

Another manifestation of Ethan's struggle to assert himself was in his developing a sleeping disorder. He was terrified to leave his mother at bedtime and woke frequently during the night. In addition, when frustrated, he had resumed biting and pulling on his mother's hair.

GRAPPLING WITH FEELING SCARED

Continuing this theme of intense reactions to transitions, in a session during this phase Ethan protested coming out of his stroller upon entering my office, all the while clutching his pack of discs. This time I too tried to use my words to engage him in talking about how scared he was. He responded by asking to write a letter and hopped out of the stroller. While dictating to me, "Dear daddy, are you at the office?" I drew the face of a "scared boy," and then a "scared boy" in a stroller. Before I could finish, Ethan demanded to dictate another letter. "Dear Dr. Sherkow, I missed you. I went to Florida. I went swimming. Airplane. I love Granny. Granny loves me." He then asked me to draw a picture of him and his grandmother holding hands. Again, we could see the neurobiological impact of a not-yet-integrated sense of self conflated with anxiety about loss during separations and transitions.

At age 32 months, more progress was demonstrated after a weekend when, upon entering my office, Ethan went directly to the pad of paper and dictated, "Dear Dr. Sherkow, I miss you on the weekend." This signified a newfound ability to create a narrative out of his experience. This was followed by new, symbolic play with Scotch tape, in which Ethan made endless streams of tape, across the lengths of the office rooms, and then from room to room, enacting the themes of separation (between rooms) and being "cut off," including fascination with "cutting" the tape. He began to eat long, cigar-shaped pretzels, and became fascinated with biting them. He tried to force the pretzels into his mother's and my mouth, calling us monsters. "Yes, Mommy and I are monster mouths!" I proclaimed. Ethan's pretend play continued as he stuffed little toys into the diaper of a baby boy doll, calling the toys "sharks." In turning passive into active, using oral regression to master his fear of losing his precious stool and penis, Ethan appeared to be enacting, on a semi-symbolic level, multiple aspects of what one might expect to find any toddler experiencing during the stage of overlap between genital discovery, toilet-training, and rapprochement.

During the next several months, Ethan's family took several trips, for which we prepared by intensive use of writing letters and making variations in our "music" to describe feelings about changes. Consequently, during the interruptions he reacted with anxiety instead of his previous artificial "stoicism." During one trip he announced several times, "Want to go home to [. . .] with Mama!" During this period, I offered the use of the bang-a-ball toy to identify a range of his feelings, in parallel to our use of musical instruments for expanding his ability to label and differentiate his emotions.

When I was about to be away for a week, we similarly prepared for the separation. Upon my return Ethan dictated, "Dear Dr. Sherkow you went away for one week. Oh no. Mom and Dad went away for four nights. Oh no. And everyone came back." Then, on another sheet of paper, "Dear Dr. Sherkow I miss you. I'm glad you are back from vacation."

Although Ethan was still "coming and going" with his discs in hand, he initiated pretend play to enact impending changes and separations, allowing us to anticipate together his dismay, fear, and worry about loss and return. Meanwhile, Ethan began to greet classmates upon entering his classroom, and, during a flight, did not need to use his CDs for comfort, nor watch a DVD, but instead played games with his parents.

At almost 34 months, upon the heels of these positive changes, Ethan's mother reported that, during his bath, Ethan suddenly stood in the tub and urinated. Developmentally, this cognitive-bodily marker signals a child's awareness of the urge to urinate. Once he can cognate that the flow of urine is about to "emerge," he stands because he wants to see his urinary stream. We speculate this marker emerges after some (unknowable) amount of time during which the child has felt this experience in its parts but now, in this moment, has "put it all together" and is excited to see the "whole" remarkable event! This marker is much clearer in raising a boy, for the obvious reason that it is harder for a parent to notice a girl urinating on herself unless she calls attention to the event. In any case, from this moment it is generally much easier to potty-train.

NARRATING CONVERSATIONS IN PRETEND PLAY

We observed something new in Ethan's next session when he pretended a Pooh Bear and Eeyore were having a conversation and included them in our little orchestra, singing to Pooh, "Hug bear very hard, very soft," (an extension of our playing the instruments very loud and very soft) and added, "No more CDs." Hugging Pooh under his chin, he said, "Huggle-snuggle bear!" and "Bear hug mama!"

Halfway through this hour, I brought up that Ethan and his family were going away for two weeks for spring vacation. His mother and I discussed the details with him: skiing, a visit to his grandparents at the beach, the number of flights, and the relatives accompanying them. Ethan then ran to the pad of paper and dictated a letter, "Dear Dr. Sherkow, I am going to ski and then to see Granny in Florida with Mommy, Daddy, [his sister], and the airplane." I then added, dictating to him, "I know you might feel worried and scared on these trips, with all of these changes, but Mommy will hug you when you are scared."

Ethan responded to this intervention by running to the block corner and inviting me to build and knock down block towers with him, an activity to which he had previously seemed averse, very afraid of the "crashing." Following a few repetitions of building and destroying towers, he picked up a baby blanket from the doll bin, lay down on my analytic couch, and snuggled the blanket under his chin, with his thumb in his mouth, for several minutes.

ACHIEVING RAPPROCHEMENT

Ethan's newfound ability to play semi-symbolically in several domains particularly in light of the upcoming vacation, seemed to have resulted from his having worked through anxiety about expressing his angry feelings to the point where he could experience a true rapprochement with his mother, allowing himself not only to be cuddled by his mother but able to represent being comforted in his play, projected onto the bear, and to represent his ability to manage angry feelings in the block play. In addition he was cognitively representing his affects in writing a letter about a potentially scary trip. His transition in the session from "aggressive" play with the blocks to snuggling with a blanket seemed to signal his newfound sense of security in his relationship with Mother and a sense of their being able to manage the upcoming transitions.

In our next hour, Ethan showed an additional developmental shift in semi-symbolic play by beginning to play with baby dolls as parent-to-baby, picking up a doll and proceeding to feed it with a bottle of water, which in turn made it "urinate." He took great delight in "making it pee," sprinkling "pee" all over the playroom floor. I simply said, "Boys like to make their penis' make pee-pee!" He responded by carrying a baby doll to the bin of Fisher-Price dolls and delightedly making the doll "pee" on the "little people," shouting, "Pee, pee!" Then, he demanded I refill the bottle, drank out of it, ran to the bathroom, grabbed lengths of toilet paper, and gleefully started flushing toilet paper, shouting, "Bye-bye pee and poo-poo!" As had happened with Johnny, there can be a moment in treatment when neuropathological symptoms have sufficiently diminished such that derivatives of previously repressed, isolated, or warded aggressive impulses suddenly emerge. What one might have expected to see emerging sequentially seems to flood the child: a profusion of fascination with body products, urinary, phallic, anal, and gender interest mingled with guilt. In our experience, this flood and the ensuing struggle to process and contain it are part of the ongoing development of super-ego and reality testing.

Ethan arrived late to his first session after vacation with symptoms of a URI. He sat contentedly on his mother's lap, sucking his thumb, and asked her to read the potty-training books. His mother laughed, recounting to me how hard she had tried during the beach half of their trip to interest Ethan in going naked. "Just go *somewhere*!" Ethan had not only refused to do so, but insisted on being given a diaper in which to urinate even when he had been wearing a bathing suit.

After listening quietly to Mom's anecdote, Ethan bounded up and started examining the bottoms of the Fisher-Price "little people," stuffing Kleenex in the hole of one of the dolls, and said, "It is peeing, like in the Joshua book!" He then put that doll on a toy potty. Next he fed a toy baby bottle to a large rubber boy doll, declaring that he was making it "pee." As before vacation, he also drank from the bottle. His mother asked him if he were going to pee too. Ethan then moved around the room, feeding himself and a host of other dolls, all of which he made "pee." Later, he ran to the dictating pad, but instead of dictating a letter drew a figure which had a shape of a body and body parts.

In our next hour Ethan asked to play baseball and for the first time was delighted at being able to strike at the balls. His mother was equally delighted and asked him if he would like to play baseball for his birthday party. He responded indirectly, picking up on her delight in his showing interest in something "boyish." "I want the boy doll," he said, but he picked up the girl doll, took a so-called "poopy" ball, and put them both in a pink blanket. Examining the doll, he discovered an inch-long red streak (made by an indelible marker) on one of the doll's legs and asked me to put a Band-Aid on it.

MENTALIZING BEING A BOY

In this exchange between mother and child, we see possible evidence of Ethan's ability to mentalize his mother's feelings and wishes, "reading her mind," imagining her thinking, "I want my Ethan to be a boy." This could have been a "compliant" reaction on his part—his announcing that he wants a boy doll seems likely to represent her wanting a boy child. Then he brought a "poopy" ball into the picture, putting it into a pink blanket. Is this defensive? In other words, was he conflicted about either complying or being boyish? Or was this further evidence, cognitively, of his gender confusion? To take this a step further, does this play represent his fantasy of his mother's hidden anal phallus? From the dynamic perspective, this bit of play does not clarify where Ethan fits developmentally but does illuminate his struggle to identify himself.

Ethan began to show additional interest in his body parts while also becoming willing to entertain the idea of toilet-training and also taking on the role of playing parent to the dolls. He sat dolls in a circle so they could listen to his mother read Sam's potty book, pointing to the page where Sam resolves his training crisis by sitting on his potty, reading a book to his dog. Then, taking down the "Joshua" toilet-training book, Ethan pointed to the pictures of the boy's penis and rectum, smiling. He then grabbed a piece of toy fruit and stuffed it into his mouth, with a devilish look in his eye, teasing us about choking. I responded, thinking that his behavior pointed to defensive anxiety about whether he was allowed to look at body part differences (picking up on the looking rather than the gender conflict) by asking if he wanted me to show him a boy doll that looked like Joshua. He agreed. I said, "He looks just like Joshua. He has a penis." Ethan examined the doll's penis and buttocks and, pointing to the doll's knee, said, "He has a boo-boo!" But, expecting to see the red mark on the doll's leg, he said, "I don't see anything there!" This was fascinating because it seemed to show all aspects of his concerns at once. Here was the boy doll, the one he asked for the day before, but not the one he had selected and hence not the one with the mark. This seemed to be denial of the genital difference. He had focused on the doll's red mark, not her "absent genital," but announced it in the presence of the "genitally intact" boy. In this context Ethan used the word "I." In the next moment, he began crashing toy cars against the wall; I joined him and together we raced cars, as he yelled "crash" for at least 10 minutes. At the end of the hour, he returned to playing with "little people," during which play he seemed to not distinguish between the boys and girls, naming a boy "a girl" and vice versa.

In the next hour, however, as Ethan continued to name boys "girls," I wondered if I should have first tried to establish his cognitive awareness of gender difference rather than jump to interpreting his defense. When he again requested to read the Joshua book, I asked him, "Joshua has a penis; do girls have penises?" "Yes." Taking an educational approach, I offered, "No, girls have something else: a vagina. Would you like me to show you a girl doll?" He responded by avoiding me altogether, running to the kitchen. That did not really answer my question. He might have been reacting to me being too pushy and directive, very different from my usual stance in following his lead, or his anxiety could be on a dynamic basis. Thus, I said, "Is this too scary?" "Yes!" he answered. Again he popped the toy fruit into his mouth, scaring us. (I didn't think to ask, "Am I being too scary?")

The phone rang, and Ethan ran to the adult office, pretending to call his father, "I miss you, I love you!" and then pretended to call his relatives. I was still trying to "read" Ethan's mind, so I pretended to dictate a letter from him to me. "Hmm. . . . Dear Dr. Sherkow, tell me, who in your family has a penis, Mommy?" "Yes," he answered. "And your sister?" I asked. "Yes," he said. At that his mother interjected and corrected him. She asked him about his father, grandfather, grandmother, and several of his female therapists. He responded accurately about all of them, until we came to me. "What about Dr. Sherkow . . . does she have a penis?" "Yes!" he said. He promptly turned to his mother and asked, "Can we go to the Thomas the Tank Engine show?"

During this phase of exploring Ethan's mind—and maybe feelings—about gender differences, Ethan's concern about things "breaking" or crashing especially came to a head one day when his apartment building's elevator broke down. For some time, Ethan had shown great anxiety about entering the elevator and often had a "meltdown" if the conditions, his CD collection particularly, were not just right. In this context, from the moment Ethan entered my office, he spent a fair amount of time trying to put his hand inside his pants but was dressed so this was physically impossible. After a while, he began grabbing his crotch instead. Then as we were dictating a letter about an upcoming alteration in our schedule, he grabbed my reading glasses and pressed them into his crotch with one hand, while scribbling "a letter" with the other. Following his lead, I added to the letter about our interruption, "Ethan is very worried about the elevator being broken at home. In fact, he is nearly hysterical about it." As I wrote, he grabbed his crotch, looking scared and bereft. "I see," I continued, "I have a feeling that when the elevator breaks, you worry that your penis will get broken too, because you are so angry at Mommy that the elevator could break."

USING THE CDS TO INTERNALIZE

It seemed this interpretation led to what was an abrupt change in the way Ethan used his CDs. Beginning with the subsequent session, instead of simply parking his CDs in his stroller until he departed, he asked to put the CDs into my CD player and actually listen to them! This transition to playing CDs offered us a shared reality and seems consistent with the concept of building joint attention, that is, mutually pointing to something we could have in common. The way he used the CDs was also interesting. As he picked up each CD to play it, he announced the composer, like a DJ, "This is Tchaikovsky, this is Bach, this is Schubert, this is 'Baby Beethoven,' this is Ella Fitzgerald." He also quickly learned the composers and categories of the music on the CDs he discovered in my office.

With great concentration Ethan would put in a disc, carefully turn on the player, find the track he wanted, adjust the volume, and look intently at me. Unsure of his expectation of me, I intuitively pretended to do what I had done when he, his mother, and I played our musical instruments, which still took place in many sessions. Playing the actual CDs seemed a logical extension of that play. Thus, in response to Ethan's stare, an implicit request for me to "do something," I began to conduct the orchestra of the first CD he had put in the player, a Mozart symphony, having no sure idea of what would follow. Ethan continued to stare at me, wide-eyed and intensely engaged, and then began to imitate my motions, mirroring my conducting and, I supposed, my facial expressions. From conducting together, him following me, we pretended to play solo instruments, violin, clarinet, and cello, all the while he very intensely gazed at me, at my eyes and at my arm movements, keeping to the rhythm of the music. His focus was entirely on resonating with me to create our replication of the music, including paying close attention to the shifts in emotion signified by the various parts of each piece.

This engagement with me heralded a long stretch of our work together in which all of the dynamics of the transference (and it truly seemed to be transference, even though his mother was present in the room) were expressed through the way he used and played the CDs. After the initial period of "taking me in" through "taking in" my reactions to and handling of the emotional quality of the music, Ethan began to be fascinated by putting those emotions into words. The music was in turn "dreamy," "scary," "exciting," or "spooky." He also labeled its nature: symphonic, clarinet, violin, cello concerto, voice, R and B, rock and roll, and jazz. He further differentiated kinds of rock and roll: the Beatles, heavy metal, etc. The expanding repertoire of differentiations within the realm of music paralleled his ability to expand his emotional, affectual repertoire, modulating his emotional and relational repertoire, translating into creating relationships that were "real," as compared to the "adorable, chatty robot" who, when destabilized, became a scary monster to his parents and family.

My sense of his play was that he was demonstrating an aspect of development that we typically can only understand by deduction: the process by which a child internalizes his parent. In this case, his analyst stood in for the parent (who was in the room) as the supportive ego apparatus that allowed for exploration of the vicissitudes of Ethan's aggression and fears of being broken and damaged by, or damaging to, his mother. Once Ethan mastered a repertoire of affects (emotions connected to thoughts and fantasies that were challenging to him, such as his fear of being abandoned by his disappointing mother) he began to experiment with the question of who was the actual identificatory object, his mother or me. He would wander around the office, retreating into his "robotic" demeanor, asking, "Is this Mommy's bicycle?" "Is this Dr. Sherkow's phone?" Who was he like, and whom did he like, were simultaneous layers beneath the question, as well as the question of being forced to choose between us: was he allowed to love me as he loved Mommy (or perhaps, at times, even more than he loved Mommy). The letters to Daddy expressing his love had always seemed, and now were more clearly understood, to perhaps express the dynamic of fearing the loss of one parent in the moment of intense pleasure with the other.

Dissecting meaning in Ethan's play with the CDs was difficult. This play suggested multiple possibilities, its complexity in keeping with his developmental surge. Did he need to choose between us, between mental representations of us that collided or were similar, that made him anxious, or did forming a more complex mental representation of us threaten his ability to individuate so that "Is this Mommy's? Is this the analyst's?" was about his struggle to understand what was his. He did not yet seem to have a mental representation of his own thoughts or feelings. Other than when we were playing music together and copying the emotions in the music, his facial expression still showed little variation, and his mood and play did not reveal a range of feelings typical for his age.

USING CREDIT CARDS TO MANAGE TRANSITIONS

At the same time as he pursued his quest of "who owns what?" and/or "who is whom?" Ethan began to involve his mother's credit cards in our work for the first time. He would take them out of her purse when he seemed to feel non-specific anxiety; one could feel increasing tension and agitation in his insistence on her giving them to him. One could only imagine that the shifts in his internal attempts to represent himself, his mother, and me as objects, and his varying emotions as acceptable, or not, to those objects, created the need for managing separations for which a baby develops a transitional object. Hence, it seemed that Ethan was actually using the credit cards at those moments of transition, calming himself by questioning his mother about what the cards were, and whose they were. In asking, "Is this Mommy's?" he was asking whether *he* was Mommy's, or possibly even if he *was* Mommy. His behavior highlighted the emergence of me-not/me and mother/analyst as "same" or "different," as he shifted to questioning how the musical phrases and the musical instruments were the same or different.

In the next weeks Ethan increasingly challenged us in his moving to become an individual. Like watching a 2-year-old testing his mother, making trial attempts to pull away and to feel empowered, to submit without becoming a victim, Ethan condensed the "terrible twos" into a few weeks! We saw this shift by virtue of the way he handled feeding the CDs into the player and choosing the tracks. He went from playing fairly large segments of the discs, focusing on internalizing the quality of the music, parallel to learning about the quality of his feelings, to testing the impact of his feelings on me by varying his method of putting discs into the player. Ethan would put a CD into the player, play a few phrases, start to enact the conducting or playing the violin, and abruptly stop the player and remove the CD. Picking up another CD, and repeating this behavior, he established a minutely configured form of play in which he could stop the machine from playing a disc just as it was about to play the track. The first time he did this, I was taken unawares and had a countertransference reaction: I felt cheated of my listening pleasure. I began to see that Ethan purposefully meant to cheat me while also damaging the CDs by abruptly removing them. He controlled me. I was his pawn as he increasingly withheld the music, exquisitely able to start and stop the player before it emitted a sound, snapping the discs in and out, and tossing them to the ground. Sometimes, he varied his control of me by putting the music on "pause!"

By now, we had accumulated 50 or so discs. During the course of the first weeks of this play, Ethan had taken his CDs out of his stroller in a loose stack of 4 to 8 discs but took great care of my CDs when extracting them from their sleeves, and immediately memorized where each had been when he first used the case, robotically commenting on any disc out of place. If a CD was missing, we knew he had taken it home, but he "played dumb," looking for it, mumbling "Baby Beethoven," which was the first disc he had lifted from me. In time he used the CDs as increasingly representational identificatory objects, like little people he missed and who would be upset with him if they were gone or scratched. He also brought in his father's, sister's, and grandparent's collections. He particularly focused on scratched discs. His mother and I tried to track whether he secretly took CDs home when he was particularly upset with one of us, but he was so surreptitious we could not be sure.

His mother and I understood that the CDs represented, in part, his manifest resistance to being toilet-trained. The CDs in their pockets were so many "poops" that he kept carefully in his rectum and/or his diaper, reflecting the verbal concern his mother had shared about his not wanting to part with his dirty diaper and demanding that she put it back on. By secretly taking my CDs home, discovered much later by his mother, he enacted both an oedipal triangle as well as his ongoing fear of losing one of us in what he enacted as an imaginary battle between mother and me for his affection.

Sibling rivalry now emerged, manifest in his stealing and bringing me his sister's DVDs. He tried to play them on my CD player, even though that was impossible. This again raised the question of a latent reference to the gender question. He had stolen her precious genital and refused to return it. Was he rendering her the victim of his hidden power (the stolen, hidden discs) to keep Mother's attention on him and not her? He also was very capable of teasing me by seriously searching my office for a disc he knew he had stolen, as consistent with the classical understanding of a boy's fantasy that a woman—mother or me—has a phallus hidden somewhere!

There was the added torture of his knowing that he had scratched a particularly favorite track of mine on a vocal CD. He would pretend that he was going to play a track he knew he had scratched, again playing dumb. At first I fell for this, but after awhile realized he was successfully getting my goat. He similarly appeared to intentionally torment us by putting on CDs that weren't music at all. He would attempt to play educational material, or DVDs he had brought that he knew we couldn't play—torture by toddler DJ!

Thus Ethan's mother and I got a good dose of how Ethan felt about being perceived as "broken" and "damaged." His ability to tease, to play dumb, and to know what was important to me suggested consolidation of aspects of his developing Theory of Mind. One interesting variation was his insistence on playing a damaged disc. "It's wobbly!" he exclaimed. Of course I heard this as an emerging metaphor: if we were going to acknowledge feelings, we three were on wobbly ground.

A feature of ensuing sessions was Ethan's preoccupation with a Paganini disc that was "born," as far as Ethan was concerned, with a scratched and unplayable track, evidence that Ethan was identifying himself as "born defective" by insisting on playing an unplayable CD. His first application of a more nuanced use of expressive language came in this context, struggling to play this "unplayable" track. "It's broken," he said, rather quietly, but without intonation, still distanced from the experience of identifying something about him we could interpret. Indeed, to have interjected at that moment, "Ethan, I think you feel broken," would have registered intellectually but not at the level of visceral feelings. I chose to wait until there was some bit of emotional connection to the idea.

IT'S BOTHERING ME: REFERENCING AN INTERNAL EXPERIENCE

Finally, Ethan extended this observation obliquely to himself, announcing, "It's bothering," several times. Here was a milestone: completely new referencing of an internal experience. After repeating himself several times, as though practicing to synthesize his inner experience with his language capacity, he said, now referring to himself in the first person, "It's bothering me."

This moment in the treatment seemed to be another example of the transforming work of therapy in the development of Ethan's cognitive and emotional connections, a moment of being in a transitional space between experiencing something outside at the same time as experiencing something inside. My hunch was borne out when, minutes later, he attacked the Paganini CD that was "bothering him" by biting it as if he were biting on his "blankie" in a moment of anger at his mother. Here again, we observed multiple layers of possible meaning. It seemed he identified in every respect with the broken CD that he worried his mother had destroyed, and conversely he was enraged that his mother thought he was "wobbly!"

Following this session, Ethan started to regularly project his feelings onto toys. In particular, he called a teddy "broken" and repaired him by covering him with Scotch tape. He also fixated on playing only the broken tracks of our CDs until I asked, "Are you practicing something that doesn't work?" Ethan responded with a play association referencing a family trip that he was now apparently processing, where his behavior had made his family very unhappy. Picking up a toy with a Mickey Mouse face, he said to his mother, as he played a track of a CD that played perfectly well, "This is Mickey Mouse Clubhouse, Mommy. It's wobbly, it's bothering." His mother responded concretely, "No, it's working." Ethan insistently replied, "This is . . . it's wobbly!"

I interjected, "Ethan, are you thinking of being at Disneyland over the holiday and feeling worried about how upset your parents were at you?"

Ethan responded, more adamantly, referring to the track, which was playing just fine, "It's bothering!" He was manifestly talking about the music. I asked again, "It's bothering you?"

Ethan replied, "This is like what we listened to in the car!" His mother confirmed, "Yes, it is like the one we listened to in the car." Ethan cleared up the mystery: he had stolen my CD and managed to secret it to the car, where they had played it over the weekend. Now I understood what bothered him. I said, "Oh, that's the wobbly part. You feel guilty about taking my CDs. How did you get them home without my seeing you?"

Ethan illuminated his anxiety about the conflation of "secret" and "damage" when he added to this play the notion of having to clean the CDs. It appeared he believed he could repair the ones that "don't work" by cleaning them. A layer of his play reflected his conflict with his mother about being toilet-trained. To some extent he perhaps felt she would be happier with him if he wasn't dirty, which was true! When I asked him how he got the stolen CDs home so secretly, his impulse to clean increased as did his determination to play a non-workable DVD on the CD player.

The metaphorical representation of this dilemma so clearly represented his mother's anxiety about how and by whom he had been damaged, and whether he was reparable. He conflated "broken, impossible, dirty, and unplayable" repeatedly in trying to clean the DVDs so as to make them work, and protested when I asked if he wanted to safeguard them by putting them in his stroller to take home. "No!" he responded. Apparently it was important to him that we confront the "the impossible" here and now!

A moment later Ethan picked up the instruments. Taking his cue, I began to sing our usual song. "No, we don't make music!" he insisted. I embraced his negativity and sang a "We Don't Make Music" version of our song to express his wish to do something that does not work.

As Ethan continued to play the unplayable CDs and DVDs, it seemed to me that he was "stuck." Again, I asked, "Are you practicing something that doesn't work? It's like our song, where we 'don't make music,' right?"

Ethan turned to his mother and again asked her to try to play the DVD. "Try it, Mommy!" She responded, empathically, "Sweetie, it's a movie. It's not music, and you know that."

"It's music!"

Mother: "It's not music." Ethan was embroiled in struggling with evidence of being irreparably damaged by and damaging to his mother.

I spoke in the language of the metaphor. "Ethan feels desperately that we need the DVD to play music." Metaphorically, this suggested I knew that Ethan knew that we all needed to believe Ethan can be "fixed." Ethan responded, giving me the answer, "We need to play Brahms."

"Yes," I said. "You can go right ahead. Let's play Brahms. Brahms works."

Ethan accepted this intervention and added a possible method of repair that related to the "toilet-training" aspect of his fear of irreparable loss and damage. He said, "I need to clean it… to clean it with the cloth." His mother congratulated him: "Good job!"

However, as is typical in an analytic therapy, we needed to go through this process multiple times—the inevitable repetition compulsion must be dealt with in order for the therapeutic lessons to sink in. Ethan began our struggle all over again by declaring, "Bach is not working!" (And of course we all knew that Bach "works.") So we repeated the discussion of his despair that something is broken. After many repetitions with different composers, Ethan, exhibiting good taste, selected the Beatles and a particular album that he knew I liked. At this point in the therapy, he was adept at reading my body language and especially understood my reluctance to stop in the middle of a song I have "gotten into."

An important step in development ensued. Ethan showed a new ability to anticipate the music that was coming. His arms poised mid-air with his pretend baton, he stared at me, ready to conduct together when the music began. His sharing with me in planning ahead, a form of joint attention, seemed to be evidence of his increased ability to read another's mind.

Yet the advance needed to be worked through from the perspective of conflict. Having achieved "joint attention" now included our joint attention toward his having stolen my CD. This invaded his ability to retain the capacity to self-regulate I had seen earlier. While putting a CD into the machine, one he considered to be a replacement for my missing CD, he must have felt a pang of guilt, because he suddenly pulled the CD out of the player and banged on the machine. I assessed he was turning passive into active, anticipating my punishing him for his theft.

I did nothing, however, other than note the aggression as he continued to put in a CD, bang on the machine, and take the disc out. He alternated this behavior with playing with a disc he had labeled "spooky" music. We had established that this music made him anxious, and I could see how he became very dysregulated by the aggression beneath the act of hurting me indirectly. He feared my retaliation. After a few minutes, he announced, "Clean it!"

The act of banging the CD player out of anger and anxiety seemed to represent a positive shift away from his compulsive hoarding or aversive behavior. I interpreted he was anxious about having lost and broken my Beethoven CD and was worried about my reaction, to which he responded by insisting, "Let's play Beatles," an offer of reparation. This speculation seemed to be confirmed by his finding "a new home tonight" for that disc.

More confirmation about Ethan linking "damage," guilt, and reparation were evident in his next play association, as he asked for the "potty" books. When his mother started to read them, he became visibly anxious, left her side, and picked up the musical instruments. Following his cue, I started to sing our "No More Potty" song, and while at first he sang along with a delighted smile on his face, he suddenly stiffened and ran to his mother's bag, asking for her credit cards.

He piled the credit cards next to his mother, and in a sing-song voice, began asking, "Is this Mommy's?" Lying on her lap, he put a credit card under his chin, snuggling with it. This was painful to watch, as it was so clear that he could not be soothed simply by her body, touch, and voice but needed the plastic transitional object in order to be comforted or reassured. Although he took the stuffed animal I offered, hoping to help him "transition" to something genuinely cuddly, he left the credit card in place. After a few minutes, Ethan picked up the baby dolls and played with their diapers and the toy potty, "pretending" to be toilet-training.

In response I pretended to be one of the dolls, singing to Ethan, "No more potty, I'm scared to go potty!" "Don't make me go potty!"

Not ready to hear his thoughts verbalized so clearly, Ethan drowned me out by playing a CD very loudly. He went back to playing with the dolls, again noticing the red streak on the leg of the girl baby doll. "She has a boo-boo. She needs a Band-Aid!" He picked up the Paganini CD from the floor and bit it. This was the disc that signified "irrevocably broken."

"You are worried someone has broken the girl doll," I said. "Maybe with their teeth."

Then, as we came near the end of the hour, Ethan ran into the analytic office and asked, "Is this Sherkow's?" about my glasses, coffee, and so on. With glee he pulled a wooden cart of alphabet blocks off of a shelf, spilling the blocks on the floor. Crouching over the pile of blocks, he pretended to urinate on them, saying "pissshhhh" as he did!

While I understood his behavior as a displacement from his struggle with his mother over toilet-training, he needed to regress to using the credit card as a concrete representation of her acceptance of him and confirmation that he still belonged to her. He needed to ask "Is this Mommy's?" before he could engage in playing at toilet-training, which was also a gift to her, embracing the idea, if not ready to comply.

SEPARATION FROM HIS PARENTS: FEELING BROKEN

In the following two weeks, as Ethan turned 37 months, he experienced a number of transitions, disruptions, and trips in his family's schedule, along with an intensification of his mother's attempt to toilet-train him. In addition, school was coming to an end, and part of their summer vacation included his parents taking a "honeymoon" trip that would last several days. They had not told their children about the trip. During their absence, Ethan became symptomatic to the extent to which he demanded to hang onto the wallets of his grandparents (for their credit cards, presumably).

During the first of our two sessions scheduled during his parents' absence, Ethan demanded I give him one of my bracelets to wear, suggesting that the bracelet reassured him just as did his mother's credit cards. During our play, he regressed to manipulating and controlling the CDs, turning passive into active. However, he newly chose to play guitar music, which he associated with his father. He concentrated on mirroring me in conducting bass guitar. He also showed a delightful reflection of our dilemma in his deciding that we should choose a CD for a "snack song." He chose the Beatles' "Come Together" and danced to its rhythm as he ate his pretzels.

Taking his cue, I brought Mommy's absence into our play with musical instruments, singing about her being away without identifying what he might be feeling. He made a play association by trapping balls inside the bang-a-ball toy. "Ah, I said, you are making Mommy be trapped inside. She can't get out!" To this he associated by using the bang-a-ball hammer to bang on the other toys as well. In another first, he also picked up Pooh Bear and stomped on him. "Oh my, Bear," I said. "Ethan is angry at you, Bear, because Mommy has gone bye-bye."

Ethan responded by saying "Hi! I'm happy!" while further stomping on the toys. I didn't know if he was denying his anger or telling me that he was happy to be expressing it.

However when he then hid "poopy balls" in a toy elevator, I perceived this as a shift into using toys in "pretend play," wherein hiding the balls represented not only hiding his poop from his mother, but hiding his mother as well. At the end of this hour, he asked to take home my replacement CD for the stolen Beethoven CD. When I suggested he take home a stuffed animal instead, to remind him of us, he insisted on taking the CD.

A day later, on the eve of his parents' return, Ethan tried to call his mother from my cellular phone. When she didn't answer, he had a pretend conversation with her and then dumped a large pile of CDs from home onto the playroom floor. As he started rifling through them, I sensed he was making conversation with me in a very real way by asking me to name and discuss the qualities of the various CDs (classical, rock and roll, etc.) even though the pattern was reminiscent of his attempting to get his mother to name all of her credit cards for concrete reassurance.

As he put a CD in the player, he intently gazed at me, waiting for me to begin conducting. "Together," he said, looking peaceful. Then, he surprised me by saying "I can't try it."

I said, "I don't understand. It's ok, you try it." Instead of playing the disc, he began naming the CDs that belonged to me. "This is Dr. Sherkow's!" I wondered if he was preoccupied with differentiating between his mother's and my belongings, or if he was asking if he belonged to me in Mother's absence. He went on to ask for new information, wanting to know exactly how many tracks there were on each CD. Taking a Schubert disc he had never played, he said "That's great music." Indeed, at this point in the session I had observed he was most engaged and connected, making eye contact, and relaxed.

However, within minutes, his mood shifted. Rifling through the CDs, he looked more and more frantic until he finally announced, falsely, "That's Baby Beethoven!" My first thoughts were that our closeness reminded him of his mother's absence or that perhaps he felt disloyal, but then I realized perhaps his guilt about stealing my CD had resurfaced. It may even have been that the guilt about the stolen CD represented the loyalty battle and underlying fear of losing me if he were no longer "broken."

Answering him, I pointed out he had taken the Beethoven disc home the day before, despite my discouragement. He banged the CD player very hard, which caused me to wonder what exactly he felt guilty about in the moment, assuming he was acting-up out of anger. When he then played the Beatles CD, I guessed that was his attempt to appease me. A few minutes later, playing a piano piece, he announced he wanted to "take this to home."

The play disruption escalated as he became insistent on controlling me by playing "non-playable" discs: medical lectures, comedy routines, and a movie. By now he had disconnected from "playing" as conversation and only wanted to know "what things are called."

Sometime into the hour Ethan asked for his graham crackers and declared we must play graham crackers music. This time he picked up one of his sister's CDs and played a song about "breaking my heart!" I saw this choice as relevant: his mother's absence and his consequent feeling of disloyalty was breaking his heart, recalling that the day before he had chosen as a snack song "Come Together!" As he ate his snack, he played his sister's "Charlotte's Web" disc, knowing exactly what we were about to hear: the part of the story (about a small, weak pig that Charlotte's father intends to kill because he "would die anyway") where Charlotte says, "Don't kill it!" to which the father replies, "Control yourself!"

Understanding the symbolism in this, I asked Ethan if he knew when his mother was coming back, to which he answered correctly that she would be returning the following day. Exchanging the book CD for his sister's Miley Cyrus disc, he sang along, familiar with the words and a special gesture from the music video. "This is the best of both worlds," he sang, seeming to have recovered from the agitation, through both reaction-formation and turning passive into active.

INTERPRETING CDS: I MISS MOMMY

Suddenly, Ethan's agitation resurfaced, and he started to pull CDs in and out of the player. Confused, I made many tries at understanding this behavior: was he having trouble deciding which one to play or worried about something not working. I asked, "Are you confused? You can't decide?" Ethan answered indirectly by increasing the rate of speed at which he put a CD into the machine and punched it out. He asked as if he wanted an answer, "Which is better?" and commented that a piano piece (one he was not playing) was "Good, great music." As he continued, I felt more flummoxed until I realized his manipulation of the discs and machine was a way of teasing and controlling me and that he was becoming rather sadistic, pulling me in to hear something with him, then shutting me out, thwarting my efforts to mirror his enthusiasm.

I felt "he isn't giving me a chance." As he continued to enact variations on the theme of thwarting us, he tossed CDs in and out of the player, slapping and hammering at the CD player multiple times, saying, finally, "That's no good!"

I began singing, "I miss Mommy. Nothing is working without her!" Ethan listened intently and hammered the floor with drumsticks following my rhythm. As long as he banged the beat, I kept singing about missing her and being "broken." I took his continuing to accompany me with his own drumsticks as encouragement to continue to invent variations such as, "The CDs make you feel like you have Mommy here." He banged the CD player, in confirmation. I went on to repeat the prior verses, leaving room in between the iterations with use of simple syllables, such as, "No, no, no, she's not." These included, "And you bang the CDs because you are angry that Mommy isn't here." "Ethan is sad because Mommy's not here." "Ethan wants to play the songs that he knows because Mommy's not here." "CDs are scary if they are very new." "Ethan likes CDs because they make him feel very safe." "Ethan is scared to be without Mommy. He takes his CDs everywhere he goes. They make him feel like Mommy is with him wherever he goes."

After at least 8 minutes of my addressing as many aspects of his dilemma as I thought he could tolerate, Ethan interrupted, "Where is baby Mozart?" He started to sing along with me, so I sang in first person, "The CDs make me feel safe. They make me feel like Mommy is here. When she isn't here, I feel like she threw me away. I feel very broken. I feel like she throws me away, it hurts my feelings!"

At that moment Ethan said "Be quiet!" and put a Brahms CD into the player. I asked him, "Should I keep singing?" "Yes," he answered.

So I resumed, "When my Mommy is not here it makes me feel broken," as he continued to play the drumsticks to the beat. Now walking around the room, he hit objects with them. After about four more minutes, I was getting weary, yet I continued until he cued me by stopping his drumming. "I want to play with the shooters!" he announced, turning to the army toys, and then threw himself into my lap.

SUMMARY

From a psychodynamic perspective, just as with ASD per se, developmental unevenness interferes with the evolution of the increasingly complex skills involved in understanding one's own and others' behavior, thoughts, and feelings. Internalizing Ethan's experience of his mother's caretaking and empathic responsiveness to his needs would have been an essential ingredient in forming representations of "experiences" between parent and child. It was fundamental to his well-being that his development consist of organized expectancies of functioning—that there would be patterns in his relationships and experiences, and that they would occur in contexts that were predictable and dependable. For Ethan, it seemed, the processes of internalization, of "taking in" the other, was especially jeopardized, leading to dysregulating his relationship to his parents. He developed a repertoire of defense mechanisms that included a rigid attachment to CDs and credit cards to manage the growing demands on him for self-regulation and integration into his family structure.

In summary, we saw in Ethan an example of developmental unevenness where an analytically based dyadic treatment was used to "catch up": to manage separation anxiety, and to resume functioning on his developmental trajectory. Using his significantly precocious auditory and musical capacities, it was possible to engage Ethan in expressing himself as he developed language for communication and became primed for mastering competencies in toilet training and authentic social relatedness. By the time Ethan was ready for kindergarten, he had evened out, with all developmental arenas on par for his age.

Chapter Five

Conclusion

In our view, dyadic treatment is not only important but essential in working with a child and his parents, whether the child has uneven development or ASD. These cases have aimed to demonstrate the extent to which intermingling of symptoms and family dynamics can be approached when working in an intimate and non-judgmental environment guided by an expert in development. Indeed, our expertise lies in assessing the normal variations in the daily presentation of the blend of a child's emotional, cognitive, and attentional experiences, both internal and interpersonal, as well as assessing where any particular day fits into the bigger picture of his relationship to his mother and his family.

Our expertise especially lies in being able to make the best possible hypothesis in "reading" a child's actions, unconventional behavior, and play enactments for their meaning. Through experience, we have learned that when we try to make the best possible sense out of a child's play or behavior, we bring attention to his "mindedness," which is of utmost importance for both the child, who needs to know that we see that he has a mind, and for his mother to see it as well. All by itself, this first step in working with a dyad takes some, if not most, of the pressure off of a child to perform, and allows underlying conflicts and ordinary negativity to emerge and be more easily addressed. In following the treatment process in our cases, we make it clear that once symptoms are accepted, understood, and then reduced, ordinary tasks of development emerge and can be confronted.

Of particular importance in dyadic work is the acceptance, from the start, of the aggressive feelings embedded in the symptom picture. Each of the children needed a way, verbally in the context of an action, to safely express their angry feelings toward their mothers in the presence of their mothers. Bang-a-ball was the most useful, as it also offered the range of emotions to be "hammered out" through the range of colors. Being able to say, "I'm angry at Mommy!" was essential to start the process of accessing emotional/cognitive processing in the three boys presented herein. This action play with aggressive content thus began correcting the parent's sense of failure in being connected to her child, and seemed as well to begin the essential integration of emotional, cognitive, and dyadic experiences. Through this new integration, we saw in each child the scaffolding of semi-symbolic and then symbolic development in language in parallel to play. These are the building blocks enabling self-regulation, reciprocal play, development of fantasy and imaginary play, and management of aggressive affect that in turn enables socialization.

Why is play so important? Play is a therapeutic action in which emotional interactions with cognitive content, or cognitive moments with emotional content, are put into action by the child. The toddlers we describe appeared to have internalized through action what they experienced in play, what Rogoff calls participatory appropriation, making meaning through joint action in the context of joint experience between child and analyst (Rogoff, 1995).

Through psychodynamically informed early intervention, it is possible to track when presenting symptoms, such as twirling or obsessive preoccupation, begin to be replaced by more typical means of expressing conflict as the child develops more evidence of ego organization, and the behavior can then be seen in use defensively. It is important to begin dyadic treatment as early as possible, ideally at the time of diagnosis, because not only does a parent obtain the support of the analyst in making meaning out of her child's dilemma, but the older the child, the more difficult it can be to manage the difficult rigidity that progressively ensues. In older children, with whom aspects of development have already become consolidated with character defense, it may become difficult to tease apart aspects of ambivalence or oppositional behavior that has become intertwined with primary ASD symptomatology. In addition, over time, the inevitable narcissistic injury arising from having a "disorder" impacts both parent and child, and becomes harder to undo.

The case material described here has also aimed to illuminate how the neurofunctional impairment in a child with ASD or uneven development can impact emerging drive derivatives and superego development as he proceeds through the psychosexual stages. The three boys described here struggled to master affects deriving from both normative development and from the disordered sense of self and of social relationships.

SOME TANTALIZING QUESTIONS

It has been postulated that children with ASD or uneven development have increased sensory responsiveness as part of their neurobiological endowment, therefore being "hyperalert" and unable to select out the kind of social-environmental input that neurotypical children use to develop social and emotional relationships (Fischbach, personal communication, 2010; Helt et al., 2008). If true, chronic states of overstimulation may then lead to social isolation or aversion on the part of the child. Symptoms such as gaze aversion may be a means of managing hypersensitivity to stimuli, which in turn they have less neuronal capacity to process. Their mother's understandable hypervigilance, anxiety, or narcissistic injury may become one such secondary source of overstimulation. In addition, a parent's ordinary anger and frustration might also be misrepresented by her child as overstimulating. In turn, we speculate that these children find concrete, non-threatening, and static replacement objects or controllable self-stimulating behaviors that are not only neutral and predictable, but perhaps even comforting.

In conclusion, we hope to lend support to the view that dyadic, psychoanalytically informed therapy remains a viable and favorable option in the treatment of ASD and uneven development. Our analytic approach holds that a positive therapeutic effect occurs through the analyst's narration and interpretation of the child's emotional and behavioral states, as compared to direct behavioral intervention. In particular, we strongly believe that a dyadic approach to treatment, in which both mother and child are active participants, is particularly advantageous.

II

Reflective Network Therapy

Chapter Six

Introduction to the Method of Reflective Network Therapy

Reflective Network Therapy (RNT), carried out in the preschool classroom by a collaboration that includes psychoanalyst, teacher, peers, other professionals such as occupational and speech therapists, and parents, is an excellent treatment option for ASD preschoolers (Kilman, 2011). The method works by building "reflective networks" for the child with the adults at school—teachers, therapists, parents—and the other children, scaffolding the developmental capacity to reflect on the connections between internal and external experience and behavior, building a "Theory of Mind" (Fonagy, Gergerly, Jurist, & Target, 2002, pp. 26–29). This reflective work occurs in multiple short (15–30 minute) psychoanalytic sessions, four or five times a week, and in the feedback sessions—between psychoanalyst and teacher, teacher and parent, analyst and speech or occupational therapist. The sessions are designed to help the children make sense of their otherwise chaotic and frightening social worlds "on the spot," making it an essentially practical therapeutic modality.

The child's school day begins with a parent briefing in which—in the presence of the child—the parent tells the teacher about events in the child's life since the end of the child's last day at school. At the beginning of the therapy session, the teacher briefs the therapist about events since the last session, including the information from the parent. The therapist uses this background plus the on-the-spot experience of the child in the classroom, in the therapeutic session. In addition to the teacher and therapist briefings, the teacher or the therapist has a meeting—either in person or on the phone—with the parents once a week, and the therapist has a meeting with the parents alone once a month. In addition to these briefings with parents and teachers, the analyst also talks regularly with the other professionals involved in the child's treatment—for example, occupational therapist, or speech therapist.

For example, the teacher finds out from the parents that the mother of a 2-year-old child with uneven development is taking a several-day trip away from the home. She communicates this to the therapist in her briefing. In the therapy session, the boy plays in the kitchen area, "cutting" pieces of play vegetables into pieces with a pretend knife. The therapist comments on the cutting into pieces and how "not good" it feels to be "in pieces" and "not together." Then the child becomes absorbed in a pretend mailbox and preoccupied with a piece of the mailbox—the flag that indicates the presence of mail—that is broken. The analyst says that the child has noticed something broken, and that she knows children do not like broken things because it reminds them of their "broken feelings." Another child joins them at this point. The analyst addresses her remarks first to her little patient and then to the other child, conscious of the value of multiple iterations offering the child many opportunities to hear and take in meanings about his world. The therapist comments that sometimes children have broken feelings when their mommies go away. The classmate replies thoughtfully, "Like I had sad feelings when my mommy went away." (This child's mother just had a baby sibling.) The analyst confirms the classmate's statement. After the session, the analyst debriefed the teacher, telling her about the child's play and how he seemed to be missing his mommy.

In another example, the mother briefed the analyst at the beginning of the school day. The mother told the analyst that her 4-year-old autistic son was talking about the end of the school year. The analyst structured some rhythmic, reciprocal play at the water table in which when the child asked her to open a tube and she made it into a game with three steps—one, two, three—open! Then the boy poured out the colored water and exclaimed, giving the analyst a sustained direct gaze and a smile, "Max made the water yellow!" and the analyst repeated, "Max made the water yellow." Adjacent to the water table, at the "goodbye window," a girl classmate started to scream and cry about her mother leaving. Max abruptly left the water table and climbed to the loft of the structure. The analyst remarked, "I think Max got scared when Andrea was crying." Max gave the analyst a direct gaze. The analyst continued, "She was crying because she didn't want her mommy to go." A little while later she added, "When a kid hears another kid crying for her mother, it reminds him that he misses his mommy too! Too many goodbyes." Max gave the analyst another direct gaze and took two pillows—one to lie on and the other to cover himself up with. The analyst remarked that Max knew how to make himself feel safe. Max snuggled into his new bed. When the analyst was debriefing the session to Max's teacher, Max jumped upright and exclaimed with alarm, "Not yet goodbyes! Not today!" The analyst and the teacher reassured him that the goodbyes were "not yet, not today." At pickup time, the teacher told the mother about the session, underscoring the meaning of "goodbyes" to this little boy. It was clear that this significantly impaired child was putting together an awareness of the end of school with separation from his mother and with feelings of loss.

This therapeutic method was designed in the mid-1960s, by child psychiatrist and analyst, Dr. Gilbert Kliman, while working with Marianne Kris and other colleagues in New York. The first therapeutic preschool service using this method opened in 1965 at The Center for Preventive Psychiatry in White Plains, New York. Originally called the Cornerstone Treatment, it later acquired the name Reflective Network Therapy in response to an increasing emphasis on the "network" of information about the child being contributed to and shared by multiple caregivers—including psychoanalytic therapist, parents, babysitter, teachers, occupational therapist, speech therapist, early intervention clinician, and so on.

One of the most attractive features of this treatment is the outcome studies that demonstrate increases in IQ and CGAS (Children's Global Assessment Scale). The first prospective study of IQ as an outcome was reported on a series of eleven consecutive RNT treatments of children in the White Plains program (Kliman, 2011, 231–280). The children in this study included three with PDD with autistic features, and others with serious emotional disorders and were tested at approximately yearly intervals from 1967 to 1978. All eleven children showed full-scale gains in IQ with an average gain of 24 points on last follow-up. In 1999, a second study of consecutive RNT treatments from 1995 through 1997 in a public school special education program in San Mateo, California, was completed (Kliman, 2011, 231–280). In this controlled study, the children treated with RNT improved significantly in both CGAS and IQ, measured by WIPPSI-R, compared with children in the control group who received excellent special education services but no psychotherapy. A particularly important finding was the increase in IQ of the treated group in direct proportion to the number of sessions of RNT the children received. Although this study had a small *n* of 9 children in the experimental and 9 in the control groups, the evaluators were blinded, and the results are promising.

RNT offers a number of advantages. In addition to the positive results in outcome studies, the method allows for the child to instantly make a more accurate and benign sense of his or her experience than many therapies more isolated from the child's everyday life. RNT does not require the child and the family to transport the child to afterschool therapy sessions in a professional office. RNT involves the parents in a vital and supportive way, and it utilizes the skills of the teachers and other therapists in an integrated approach to the child's treatment. Furthermore, the therapy is highly cost effective in that the analyst sees the child in fractions of a session multiple times a week, which allows for the sessions to be billed as 15- or 25-minute psychotherapy sessions, according to the new CPT coding criteria. Thus, RNT offers the child and family the possibility of a high frequency of therapeutic sessions in combination with an intense involvement in the fabric of the child's relational and educational life, at a fraction of the cost, and without extracting the child from his or her daily routine.

Chapter Seven

Dahlia

I met the little girl I call "Dahlia" when she was 3 years old. Shortly after the treatment began, Dahlia received psychological testing and was given a diagnosis of autism. After a year and a half of treatment, she was retested and had lost this diagnosis. Following preschool, she was accepted at an independent school for typical children and has done well, although she continues to be somewhat constrained in her interests and choice of friends, and she sometimes has difficulty complying with classroom directions that are challenging or confusing to her. She has exceptional artistic talent and is a beautiful child. This is the story of her evaluation and the early years of her treatment.

REFERRAL

Dahlia was referred to me because of her parents' concerns that her "development was not normal." Her parents described her as "hard to reach" and "lacking emotion and empathy," and they were worried that she was autistic. The teacher in her preschool classroom described her as unresponsive to adult direction, as uninvolved with her peers, and as sometimes behaving in bizarre and even dangerous ways in the classroom, such as climbing on furniture. In addition, Dahlia had difficulty with transitions both at home and in the classroom. She would often seem to ignore or not to hear cues about the need to stop what she was doing and move to another place or another task, and when an adult would insist on this move, it could provoke a tantrum.

I obtained the following family history from Dahlia's parents. Both parents were born in Asia and at the time of the referral were in their late thirties. Dahlia's mother immigrated in grade school, and her father in late adolescence. Her mother has a BA and held a professional job, and her father had a post-graduate degree and worked in an IT company. There was family history for left-handedness, and autism. Mother's brother had an autistic son, and mother had a cousin with autistic characteristics. Both father's parents were physicists, and father's sister and mother were both considered to have difficulty in social relationships. In addition, father's family experienced traumatic separations during the cultural revolution.

Dahlia's parents then reported her developmental history. There was a great deal of pressure on both sides of the family to have a child. Dahlia was born after a normal pregnancy, and was cared for primarily by her mother but also to a significant degree, by her maternal grandmother, who lived in the same city. At 10 days old, Dahlia was admitted to the hospital because of jaundice. Her mother had first noted "low energy." The baby stayed in the hospital for one day. At 2 months old, Dahlia's mother became concerned that she had little eye contact with her baby and the baby was not playful or interactive. Yet, Dahlia's milestones seemed normal; she walked at 1 year, spoke her first words in Mandarin at 12 months, and was joining words into sentences at 18 months.

However, as a toddler, Dahlia was not interested in other children or dolls. Instead, she played with flowers and fed them as if they were her babies. She knew the names of the basic emotions but not the subtle ones, and she could not name her own emotions. Dahlia seemed sometimes not to know whether she was hungry or cold. She would have to be told to put on her coat and mittens even when it was very cold outside. She also would not notice the need to empty her bladder until the last minute and would need to be reminded to go to the bathroom.

Dahlia entered preschool at 2-1/2 years old speaking only Mandarin. Contrary to the expectations of her parents and of her teachers, Dahlia did not learn to speak English. Her parents wondered whether this was because she was having trouble making a transition from Mandarin or whether she had a "primary language problem." At this time she began repeating scripts from videos. She remained isolated from her peers. The following year her parents transferred Dahlia to a different preschool, where I consult, and in November she was referred to me for evaluation.

EVALUATION SESSION AT 3 YEARS OLD

The evaluation session was videotaped, according to my usual way of working. The unusual degree of detail presented in this account taken from an analysis of the videotape is offered as an illustration of the behavior of a child with ASD and her family interactions. The observations drawn from videotape demonstrate both the common features of children with ASD and also the uniqueness of each child with this diagnosis.

Family Observation

When Dahlia and her family entered the room for the evaluation session, the first observation I made was of her expressionless face with big, dark eyes. First I asked her father to play with her. Her father got down on the floor and expressed his wish to play with her, but Dahlia moved around so that her back was to him. Her father then got up and walked around so that he could sit facing her. They had a conversation about a toy boat. Father's pace was slow and measured. Dahlia asked, "Why doesn't it move?" Father explained, reaching into the basket and taking out a toy car, "You need some kind of car to tow it." Dahlia responded with a negative tone, "This doesn't have any car to tow it," as if her father's remark were an intrusion. Father quietly repeated Dahlia's response. Father then introduced a person into the play. "Do you want someone to sit inside and drive it?" he asked. "Otherwise it has no driver." Dahlia quickly answered, "I don't want . . . I can drive like this," running the car along the floor back and forth. Father responded, "Okay, you can drive like this." He then shifted his weight in the sitting position so that his torso and head moved way back, before regaining his original posture.

I then asked Mother and Father to "change partners," so that Mother would play with Dahlia. The parents exchanged their position in the play area without a word. Dahlia did not look up at all during the exchange and murmured quietly to herself.

As her mother approached her, Dahlia gave her a brief direct gaze of hypervigilance and then averted her gaze, turning her head away. Her mother reached into the play space to gesture toward the dinosaur scene that Dahlia had set out, while Dahlia turned away to reach for a block in another basket with her right arm. In this movement, her left arm made an incomprehensible up and down movement that resembled the "swimming" movements sometimes pointed out in strange situation examples of "disorganized attachment" but also could have signified the fending off of an intrusion. As Dahlia moved her hand holding the block back into the play space, Mother withdrew her arm and sat back, placing the same hand under her chin in a pensive, and also, functionally, a respectful, gesture.

Dahlia stated that she was building a house for dinosaurs. Mother asked her many questions, and Dahlia answered all of them, but over time she expressed increasing negativity. "Is that a door?" Mother asked. "No, that is not a door. I don't want the dinosaurs to get out," Dahlia responded testily. Mother's positive affect was intense and her pace fast. When Father joined them, as I asked him to do, neither Dahlia nor her mother made an explicit response to his presence. Both parents were highly attentive to Dahlia. She looked overwhelmed, as her parents commented on her building and began to add some blocks to her structure.

My Play Evaluation of Dahlia

When I asked her parents to allow Dahlia a moment to play alone before I got down to play with her, they left her without explanation, and she again did not look up to acknowledge their departure. Her gaze averted, she murmured quietly to herself. I sat down near her, and she gave me an initial direct gaze and then referenced her parents in a quick glance. Dahlia told me that she was making a house for dinosaurs. I made an initial affirmative, "Mm Mm." Then the videotape demonstrates a series of gestures in which Dahlia and I made an enhanced connection. Dahlia knocked something over, and as she withdrew her hand, my hand moved slowly forward. I retrieved the fallen block very slowly. Dahlia took the block from my extended hand, and I left my hand in the offering position for a quarter of a second (a long time), waiting for Dahlia to withdraw her hand before I withdrew mine. I asked Dahlia if she would like more help in picking up blocks that had fallen down, and she said yes. Again, my moves were slow and steady in retrieving the fallen blocks. As she sat back from the finished dinosaur house, she gave me a direct gaze and said, "Mm." I then repeated "Mm," 1/10 second later. When the videotape was analyzed, the timing of our joint "Mm" . . . "Mm" is exactly the same as the "Mm . . . Mm" of my original affirmation to Dahlia. This expression of high attunement in the nonverbal domain of communication set the tone for our future relationship.

Viewing the Video with Parents

In the clips with Father, I noted the positive features of his slow, predictable pace—similar to Dahlia's—and his ability to follow her lead in the play. In that context, I asked him about his suggestion of a doll for her play with the trailer. He said that he wanted her to introduce people into her play because of his worry that she was autistic. When I pointed out his backward swaying movement, he explained sadly that he had felt rejected when she firmly declined his offer.

In the clips with Mother, I pointed out her many affirmative responses to Dahlia and her wide range of affect, how she offered ideas to help Dahlia elaborate her play, and how hard she worked to engage her. Then I pointed out Mother's "mismatch" behavior—the intensity of her affect and her fast pace. I asked Mother's intention, and she responded, "To connect with her." I asked Mother's feelings, and she responded, "Rejected, sadness," then added, "It was for me," indicating that she understood her behavior had been motivated by her own needs rather than those of her daughter. At that point I showed them what I called the "repair pattern"—when Mother withdrew her hand, sat back, and put her hand under chin, in an implicit invitation for Dahlia to "take a turn" or "hold the floor," a counter move against intrusion. I explained that every time one of her parents repeated a similar "repair," they built hope for something better in the future. In the clip of Dahlia playing with me, I showed them the moment when she referenced them when I approached her for the first time; that demonstrated their importance to her and the way she looked to them as a source of safety when threatened. I also demonstrated to them her pretend play skills and indicated to them that this was also a hopeful sign.

COMMON OBSERVATIONS IN ASD FAMILIES

A number of features of autism and of the experience of having an autistic child were illustrated in my review of the tape with Dahlia's parents. Their feelings of sadness and rejection when their child withdrew from them and declined their invitations for engagement are common to most parents of children with ASD. These feelings were demonstrated by two of Dahlia's father's movements. First, he shifted his position so that he could face her instead of having her back to him. Next, he rocked backwards in his seated position when she declared that she didn't "need anyone to drive it." Dahlia's mother indicated similar feelings in reaction to Dahlia's lack of interest in her approach and in her invitation to play with her.

Dahlia's family demonstrated common behavior patterns that may inhibit the potential growth of an ASD child's developmental capacities. Her parents tended to intrude into her space and her activity when Dahlia did not include them. Then, when she reacted negatively to their intrusion, her father initially seemed to give up. This problematic pattern of mismatch in the relationship between parent and child is common in the families of ASD children and results both from the difficulty in "reading" the child's feelings and intentions and also the parents' lack of strategies for engaging the child. The defensive withdrawal on the part of parents and other caregivers works against the development of the social skills of communication and reciprocity, and the capacity for enjoyment of other people, that these children so desperately need. A more felicitous set of responses might be to identify Dahlia's focus of attention, join it, and then in a step-by-step way, help her move her agenda forward, in this case, exploring the toy basket or building a dinosaur house. If the child withdraws, the parent can gently insist on engagement instead of withdrawing him- or herself in response to the perceived rejection.

Also, it is likely that the parents' anticipation of Dahlia's lack of recognition of their comings and goings implicitly influenced their failure to verbally prepare her for transitions. A more helpful approach might have been to talk her through the transitions: "Now I am going to sit down and keep you company while Mommy plays with you!" or "Now Dr. H is going to play with you and Mommy and Daddy are going to sit over here." Especially if delivered with strong positive affect, these remarks can become part of the guiding framework of Dahlia's daily routine.

Dahlia's parents also seemed to misread her quiet, self-regulatory murmuring to herself as contentment. With the awareness that this might instead be an indication of stress, they were better prepared to respond empathically. It was clear to me that these potentially inhibiting behaviors represented only a part of the repertoire of the relational patterns in the family. In addition, the family possessed many positive parenting behaviors. I was impressed and gratified to hear from Dahlia's mother in the last meeting of the evaluation that she had noticed several behaviors of mine when I was playing with Dahlia—my slow pace, my staying close to Dahlia's agenda, and my narrating Dahlia's play—that she had already started to reproduce in play sessions with Dahlia at home.

In fact, another common problematic pattern in families of ASD children is conflict between the parents with the child as the focus. If the father continually withdraws from interactions with the child, the mother will often move into a dominant protective role, resulting in the father being further excluded. The mother becomes the only parent who "understands" the child. The relationship between the child and the mother becomes increasingly exclusive in the family and opportunities for a strong positive relationship with the father diminish. In addition, the mother can become overwhelmed with responsibility for the child—the complex and multiple therapeutic arrangements—and become resentful at her husband's freedom from this burden.

PLAN FOR TREATMENT

I confirmed Dahlia's parents' concern that she had ASD, while also emphasizing the positive potential for her future growth and development and acknowledging the uniqueness of every "ASD" individual. We brainstormed what they wanted to do and they accepted my recommendation to treat Dahlia 4 to 5 times per week and for them to meet with me regularly in parent consultation. Since I already worked in Dahlia's preschool, it was agreed that I would see her 3 to 4 times a week in the preschool and once in my home office. I included the once-a-week office session because this was my first attempt at RNT and at that point I felt more comfortable working in an office setting. By the end of the first year, my comfort and confidence in the preschool work had grown to the degree that I felt I no longer needed an office session, but I kept it in place because the treatment was working well. In the third year of treatment Dahlia graduated from the preschool, and all the treatment was conducted in my office.

FIRST YEAR OF DAHLIA'S TREATMENT

My work with Dahlia in the classroom followed the Reflective Network Therapy method of treating ASD children, a psychoanalytic method of treating children with serious psychological disorders in the preschool classroom (see chapter 6). In my office, I used my standard method of psychoanalytic play therapy. Dahlia's parents and I met infrequently, but her mother joined a mother's group for mothers of "quirky kids" that met weekly. In the group, which I co-led with a DIR-trained occupational therapist, the mothers brought videos of themselves playing with their children and the group gave them feedback. I will include a couple of examples of Dahlia's mother's contributions in this account.

In my early work with Dahlia, I spoke and moved my body in simple, repetitive actions to establish rhythms that were predictable and could communicate security. I was careful to position myself opposite her so that if she did gaze at me directly she could see my face. I used my face and voice to express affect in an amplified manner. I was careful to follow her lead in the play, and I looked for opportunities to support her initiative.

In the first session in the office, Dahlia chose to play with the dinosaurs and told me about a movie about dinosaurs in which a dinosaur broke his horn when he was in a fight. I remarked that it sounded like a scary movie, but Dahlia denied that this was the case. She pointed out an elephant with a broken tusk and then said that she was finished with playing. I said that lots of kids didn't like broken things because it gave them broken feelings. She returned to the play and started sorting the dinosaurs into bigger and smaller dinos. She said that I could have the small dinos and she would keep the big ones. I said that when things were broken and scary it was good to be big and strong. Dahlia then worked to connect a small truck cab with its trailer and succeeded. After that, she found a manger and tried to make a small animal drink from it; when it could not reach, she created a step from a block so that the animal could reach.

In this session, as in the ones that followed, I worked consciously in multiple domains—attending to her state of regulation, watching out for her initiative, and also, as she introduced it, following the familiar theme of the dangers of aggressive power. In addition, I wondered if her connecting the trailer was a reference to another related theme of "repair of ruptures." I had identified this theme in the family meeting. Perhaps this theme was also represented in the creation of a step up to the trough so the baby animal could drink. I thought that a fear of rupture in the mother-child relationship would naturally follow the representation of destructive aggression. Her creative solution to the high trough previewed a creative capacity that would emerge in greater degree as we continued.

These conflictual themes are not unusual in my experience with neurotypical children—especially conflicts about aggression. What became clearer in my mind as a distinction between the play with Dahlia and the play with other young children was the paramount need to support her fragile regulatory functions, and the challenge to engage her in an affective, reciprocal interaction with me that moved forward toward greater complexity in the play instead of getting stuck.

In the office Dahlia and I continued to play with the dinosaurs. I discovered that she "did not like elephants," but although I had many ideas of why she disliked them, I could not get her to confirm any of them. The play was enjoyable to me, but it soon became clear that the creativity evident in the first session was not often available to her. Instead, she regularly set forth a scenario of dinosaurs and farm animals. The dinosaurs were good and the farm animals were bad, especially the pigs. As the play went on, the goal of creating reciprocal exchanges and of moving her rigid positions toward greater flexibility grew increasingly important.

In the classroom, Dahlia was at first an outlier in the group of neurotypical peers. No one disliked her, but at first no one could be identified as her particular friend. Yet, Dahlia maintained a lively interest in her classmates and was extremely responsive to their communications to her. One day at circle time, her teacher was beginning a book that featured an elephant. Dahlia shouted, "No! I don't like elephants!" The teacher tried to ascertain the reason why Dahlia didn't like elephants and to suggest alternative ways of managing her antipathy other than prohibiting the class from enjoying this book. None of this worked with Dahlia, who continued to scream. Then a boy sitting next to Dahlia said in a matter of fact voice, "Dahlia, we know you don't like elephants. You don't have to say it again and again." Dahlia looked at him and closed her mouth. She covered her ears but allowed the book to be read.

In my office, Dahlia continued to play "good guy/bad guy" themes. Although she usually preferred to use dinosaurs as the characters in the play, sometimes she used vehicles, such as a bulldozer. One of my goals was to help Dahlia "grow" her play so that it became less routinized and more open to creative elaboration.

An example of how I worked with Dahlia in this way was when she set up the scenario on my library ladder steps, with the bad guys occupying the two top steps and the good guys entering from the surrounding area and attacking them. I asked, "What did the bad guys do to make them bad?" She responded, "I don't know. Let's play." My question was repeated multiple times with the same answer, until one day I told Dahlia that I was not going to continue the play until she helped me to understand what "my" bad guys (she always demanded that I play the bad guys) had done to deserve punishment. She responded that they ate the good guys' food. We then were able to represent this greater complexity in the play in which the bad guys noticed the good guys' food, plotted to steal it, stole it and began to eat it, and were attacked by the good guys, who retrieved their food, leaving the bad guys hungry again. Dahlia offered a further elaboration when I made a crying sound for one of the bad guys after his food was taken away. She said that my bad guys could have food, just not *that* food. She then gave them a substitute for the good guys' delicious apples they had originally coveted.

The rhythm of the play still included lots of repetition, but incremental elaborations brought us forward. The bad guys started to trick the good guys by pretending that they were not going to take their food after all, but were only offering to keep an eye on it while the good guys went on a little trip. Later, when the good guys took back their fruit, they gave the bad guys fruit trees to grow their own fruit. And so on. At the same time as the narrative became increasingly complex—though still without the fluid improvisational quality of a neurotypical child—Dahlia and I worked on naming the affect states that were generated in the play and regulating them together through attuned rhythmic exchanges.

Transitions in the play were another focus of therapeutic attention. Whereas Dahlia typically insisted on controlling the play, and I allowed her to do this to a significant degree, I did not let Dahlia control the end of the session. I addressed her attempts to do so by giving her predictable warnings and then talking to her about how hard it was to stop, while I was easing her out of the room. I told her that I understood that *she* believed she absolutely needed to complete the very last detail of her project and to leave right away felt interrupted, even "broken." However, I said, we needed to stop when I said our time was over, and she and I would work on making her strong enough to manage her big feelings about stopping.

MOTHERS' GROUP

In the first year of treatment, Dahlia's mother attended a mother's group for "quirky children" that I co-led with a DIR-trained occupational therapist (FN). Dahlia's mother quickly picked up competence in analyzing videotapes and made astute but always tactful, observations of the other participants' tapes. In one tape that she brought in of her own interactions with Dahlia, she showed how she was able to engage Dahlia in cleaning up her toys by making it into a game instead of a struggle. The other mothers were very impressed. In another tape, she showed how she helped Dahlia finish a hike after complaining she could not do it and threatening to sit down on the trail. Her method was to direct Dahlia's attention to various flowers and plants along the trail and making up stories with her about them. Dahlia's mother's capacity to invest herself in coming to know her daughter in a profound way and in advocating for her in school was proving to be a major asset in Dahlia's growth and improvement.

At the end of this year, Dahlia's neuropsychological testing resulted in the loss of her diagnosis of autism. At this point, she not only played with dinosaurs, but also with other toys, including a doll—though dinosaurs still figured prominently. The play themes continued to represent prototypical battles of virtues and vices, of good and evil. She demonstrated an intense attraction to aggressive experience. In the play, she expressed conflict in response to her fear of loss as a result of aggressive confrontations, rather than demonstrating more clearly evolved conflict, that is, fear of retaliation.

Yet, many features of her initial presentation were recognizable, such as her difficulty keeping up with the constantly shifting themes and actions in the play of her peer group, and a continuing rigidity in cognitive style. The latter was especially prominent when she was stressed. When comfortable, she could usually move into the intermediate territory between good and bad, black and white. She remained a perfectionist and would often get distressed to the point of getting overwhelmed if something she was making wasn't just right.

COLLABORATION WITH OTHER PROFESSIONALS

During the first year of treatment, Dahlia's parents engaged the services of an occupational therapist trained in the DIR ("floor time") method, and also of a speech therapist. Both therapists also used the medium of play in their work with Dahlia. The occupational therapist came to the school, where she was able to work on supporting the growth of Dahlia's body strength, coordination, and sensory integration, as well as the continuing development of pretend play, and the speech therapist worked on Dahlia's pragmatic speech in the context of her play with peers. For a period of time, Dahlia attended a small playgroup run by both these therapists. Communication with these therapists occurred in telephone calls, "corridor consultations" at the school, and in occasional "team meetings" organized by Dahlia's mother. Collaboration with them increased my knowledge of the various means by which children with ASD could be supported in their healthy development. This collaboration also offered me the opportunity to explore the way body and mind were inextricably linked in the understanding and treatment of developmental problems. I have continued to work with therapists from these disciplines and have learned a great deal about how to understand these children and how to incorporate techniques—especially methods of supporting regulation of motor activity and arousal state—into my therapeutic repertoire.

SECOND YEAR OF TREATMENT

Dahlia was playing in the playground with buckets of "found objects." Spying another bucket, she grabbed it up, without pausing to check out the circumstances of its current use. In fact, that bucket had been the centerpiece of an elaborate play about hidden treasures being carried out by a small troop of boys. When suddenly they discovered their bucket to have been appropriated, they became outraged and "told on" Dahlia to the teacher. I moved in, preparing to help with the negotiation, but it turned out that my help was not immediately necessary.

After voicing their complaint, the teacher calmly asked Dahlia if she knew that the boys had been using the bucket. Dahlia was looking stunned, her face blank. After a moment's silence, another of the boys ventured, "Maybe she didn't know we were using the bucket." A third boy added, "Maybe she thought it was just a bucket." A fourth boy said, "Yeah, maybe she didn't know there was treasure inside." It was an orchestral pattern of communication, with little phrases emerging from different locations in the group, separated by pauses. Dahlia glanced at each of the speakers, taking in what she could of their clear, age-appropriate statements.

After the bucket had been restored to its rightful owners, I had a chance to slowly, bit by bit, repeat the essence of the communication to Dahlia. The whole experience was made more intelligible by the source of information being her peers and by the gentle repetitive quality of the exchange. My psychoanalytic understanding of Dahlia's inner world—the compelling quality of her desires, her frequent obliviousness to the world of other subjectivities, and the rigidity of her cognitive processes—was essential in my intervention and non-intervention.

Another example on the playground occurred when Dahlia had been playing with her "best (only) friend," Frannie. They were playing dinosaur family. A group of other girls in their class came up to them and, when they found out what they were playing, wanted to join in. Soon one of them suggested that the dinosaur family have a birthday party. Another girl enthusiastically exclaimed that she could run and get the "birthday cake" (a playground toy); another ran to get the "candles" (some twigs). The happy hubbub surrounded Dahlia and Frannie. Then, just as suddenly as they arrived, one of the new girls proclaimed, "Look! There is a tornado coming! Quick! Run away! Run away!" and they all ran away, Frannie included, leaving Dahlia alone.

I moved to her side, preparing to say something about her feelings about what had just happened. Instead, she asked me, "What is a tornado?" I decided to respond literally and said, "A tornado is a big, black cloud of wind that comes out of the sky and is so strong that it can blow things to bits!" Dahlia looked satisfied with this explanation. She glanced around to see that two younger girls from another classroom had sat down on the bench behind her and were engaged in conversation. She addressed them, "Look!" she exclaimed. "There is a tornado coming! Quick! Run away! Run away!" The littler girls looked up at her, squealed, and ran away, giggling. Later, I heard her repeating my explanation of a tornado to a teacher. This example hints at the complexity of treating ASD children. Could I have made an interpretation about Dahlia's feelings about being left alone by Frannie and the other girls? Could I have interpreted something about the dangers of aggression inherent in the representation of the tornado? Yes, I could have. On the other hand, meeting Dahlia exactly where she was in her thinking, giving her the information that could allow her to have a meaningful social experience, one that might repair the hurt of the earlier abandonment, was the alternative I chose. Tornados turned up as a destructive aggressive theme in our play therapy later on.

In my individual sessions with Dahlia, the dynamic theme of *aggressive* power continued to dominate our play. Her conflict about aggression was demonstrated in her attraction to the T. Rex on the one hand, while on the other, her identification of plant-eating dinosaurs and jungle animals as "broken," weak, and defective. Often, she would follow one of these characterizations of a broken or defective animal with a play interruption, for example, anxiously pointing out the broken leg of one of my animals. In this play, I understood her to be representing dangerous—associated with anger, and incipiently out of control—aggression as she experienced it inside herself. She felt conflict because the aggression was directed toward her parents, whom she depended on to keep her safe. Also, she feared the aggression she perceived in her parents' faces and voices when they lapsed in their empathy for her and became disappointed and frustrated at her noncompliance or temper outbursts.

As mentioned, one of my goals was to help Dahlia "grow" her play so that it became less routinized and more open to creative elaboration. Dahlia still tended to stick to one play scenario and repeat it every session with little observable variation. What made this particularly problematic was that the narrative was reductive. The story basically involved the good guys attacking the bad guys with growls and yells. There was no explanation of what the bad guys did to make them deserve such an attack and no explanation of how the punishment was chosen or even planned out. Only at my quiet but firm insistence did some of these questions get answered.

An example of how these goals were approached is seen in a series of sessions at the beginning of the second year of therapy—in "bad guy" play. In this play, repetitive, rhythmic coordinated patterns of voice and action were established between Dahlia and me, as we played out the same story again and again with small variations on the theme until there was a resolution. There were good guys, played by Dahlia, and bad guys, played by me. The symbolic content of the conflict we played out was that between good and evil, desires and prohibitions against taking what you want right now, even if it doesn't belong to you. Played out on a library ladder in my office, with the her good guys (dinosaur figures) set up on a higher rung and my bad guys (less desirable dinosaur figures) on a lower rung, the action always played out the same way. The good guys had food that the bad guys desired, and the bad guys tried to steal it from the good guys. The robbery transpired quickly, leading almost immediately to the fierce retaliation by the good guys in which the bad guys were triumphantly demolished.

Using the voices of my bad guys, I gently objected to the pace of the battle, explaining that I wanted a chance to think about the robbery first, to plan it, and—especially—to understand what my motivation was in the first place. Grudgingly, Dahlia agreed, and with her responses to my guesses or questions about the bad guys, a fuller picture was created. I say "created" instead of "emerged" because I do not think that Dahlia had this more complex story in her head to begin with; creating the complexity was part of the therapeutic action. It turned out that the good guys had delicious fruits (cherries, apples, pears) because they "worked for it," but the bad guys, who were lazy and refused to do things they didn't want to do, had no food. Actually, the bad guys were not real planners. Rather, they observed the good guys enjoying their cherries and the idea of delicious cherries popped into their heads and they right then had to have those cherries! You can imagine what was going through my mind at Dahlia's characterization of the bad guys! The picture in my head was even more vivid due to my experiences with Dahlia on the playground and in the classroom during the rest of the week. Because of my observations of Dahlia outside the office, I was able to use some of her words and phrasing from these other contexts for the bad guy talk, without having to confront her with a direct interpretation.

The aggressive theme here is obvious, but what about the themes of reparation and "intermediate." The "intermediate" position appeared when, one day, Dahlia's good guys thought up an ingenious way to really be "good guys" but still get back at the bad guys for their previous transgressions. They gave them fruit that at first glance looked perfectly fresh but actually was rotten and disgusting. After having gobbled down the rotten fruit and having expressed the appropriate revulsion, much to Dahlia's delight, I made my bad guys protest, "Hey! Giving us rotten fruit was not exactly a 'good guy' thing to do!" Dahlia was at first stumped, and when she was stumped, she became irritable. She tried to get away from this obvious contradiction, but my bad guys held firm in their objection. Finally, she made her good guys say, thoughtfully, "Well, I guess good guys can't be good all the time, and bad guys also aren't bad all the time. Sometimes guys are kind of in between." As a matter of fact, for the first time there was a real reunion, as the good guys and bad guys danced around, singing, "We love being bad guys! We love being bad guys!" At the end of this session, the good guys and bad guys had made a tentative truce—a repair following this new insight about an intermediate position. However, this was just one step in a long series of battles of good and evil. Insights in this kind of work are not solitary achievements; rather, they have to be created and recreated again and again in this context and that, until a new territory of greater complexity and flexibility is organized in the child's mind.

In our sessions, another powerful theme appeared: of *reparation*. Although I usually think of efforts at repair as being defensive, in Dahlia's case it seemed more complicated. Alongside the broken and defective, there often seemed to be a representation of the potential for repair. Perhaps I noticed this because of the image of Mother sitting back and putting her hand respectfully under her chin in the initial family video. Whenever the theme emerged, I tended to understand it as a complex communication—partly a wish to undo or avoid the aggressive theme, and partly a hopeful wish for the future.

The third important theme I could identify was that of an "*intermediate position*." Especially in my work with preschool children, but actually in all my therapies, I look for "in between" as a welcome increase in complexity that points the direction out of a rigid, stuck solution (Harrison & Tronick, 2011). In my work with children with ASD, their characteristic rigidity requires repeating or "practicing" the creation of an intermediate solution in an effort to build a new competency. This rigidity also plays a central role in transitions. In order to make a change, move one's body to another space or pay attention to another task, a person is required to take apart his current state of organization (in multiple domains) while putting together another organization—of attention, motor activity, etc. This set of transactions takes energy for anyone, but for children with ASD or uneven development, it can feel overwhelming. Careful scaffolding of the child in the moment, plus thorough discussions with other caregivers about the issue, can work toward "growing flexibility," as I explain it to my child patients.

At the beginning of the third year into the analytic treatment, Dahlia had expanded her repertoire and not only played with dinos, but also with other toys, although dinos still figured prominently. The theme of the play remained the prototypical battle of good and evil. In one session, Dahlia made an interpretation of her own, linking what was happening in the play, with her difficulties at school.

We were playing with cars. As usual, we began by dividing up the cars into good guy and bad guy teams. Also as usual, Dahlia was behaving in a highly controlling way toward me. This is something I usually didn't mind, but on this day my back was hurting me and I was feeling a little vulnerable. Dahlia was hard at work, depositing all the good guy cars close to where I was seated (rather stiffly) and the bad guys, which I was supposed to play, on the far side of the car case away, from me. I suggested that we move the good guys over to the other side, closer to her. She objected, telling me that *I* should move, as if this were an entirely reasonable solution. I was thinking that I was not going to like what was about to happen. I was also thinking that what I was not going to like is also what her peers and teachers do not like about being with Dahlia. I assessed the affective tone of the relationship and Dahlia's regulatory status, as I considered asserting myself in a new way in the play, creating an innovation. I knew that this would dysregulate her and that I was going to create a perturbation in our dyadic system. I was hoping that the result would be an emergent property.

I declined to move, and for the moment, the confrontation was averted, as Dahlia continued her explanation of the guys. I noted that her cognitive and attentional rigidity interfered with the flow of information she received. She did not notice my refusal to move, because it was new. I had never asserted myself against her control in this way before. She told me that there was one car that was "in the middle" and neither good nor bad. I was very interested in this "middle position," of course, since it indicated to me an increase in complexity, away from the polarization and simplicity that often characterized her play. I remembered the dino game of the rotten fruit.

Dahlia set up a "fence" that was a "trap" between the good guys and bad guys. She again told me to move. I did not move. She looked confused; why was I not following directions? I stayed put. She got mad. I told her that people don't like to always have to follow her rules. I continued, reminding her that I had asked her to change the order of the good guys and the bad guys multiple times and that she hadn't listened. She averted her gaze and whispered, "That happens to me all the time." I acknowledged this was true and told her that it was good she noticed that because knowing something is the first step toward change. She mentioned the "middle" car, and I suggested that if any of the cars could change, it would be that one, because that one was already "in the middle." She agreed.

Would Dahlia have responded to my assertiveness if I had not allowed her to control me hundreds of times before, establishing a pattern of security in our relationship, given the constraints of my freedom? How much was my behavior, and thus the pattern of control she and I constructed previous to this session, related to a transference configuration derived from Dahlia's family relationships? Which was the "enactment"—the assertive behavior in this session, or the consistent pattern of control and constraint previous to my challenge? How could I use the information gained from these insights to support Dahlia's continuing development at home, in school, and in my office? I do not know the answers to these questions definitively. I do know that I used the insights gained from her sessions in my office and in the school to inform her parents, teachers, and other professionals involved in her care about what was going on in Dahlia's mind so that all the important people in her life could grow, with Dahlia, in their understanding and acceptance of her, and in their capacity to support her in her further development.

CONCLUSION

The case of Dahlia is an example of the way I work with an ASD child. I learned a great deal from Dahlia, and from her excellent parents. The themes of aggression, reparation, and in between continued to be familiar psychodynamic themes both in my work with Dahlia and with other children. They have for me a particular significance, however, in the case of ASD. That is because aggression always seems more dangerous when you start out feeling incipiently out of control, repair of a rupture in a relationship is always harder to accomplish when the relationship itself so often presents a threat, and an intermediate position is a great challenge when you see the world in polarized terms. Working on all those themes in multiple contexts and venues builds flexibility and adaptability.

III

Neurobiology and Psychoanalysis

Chapter Eight

Neurobiology, Neuroplasticity, and Psychoanalytic Treatment

William M. Singletary, MD

> . . . as so often is the case when two approaches provide different angles on the same, complex question—joining forces can be beneficial to everyone.
>
> —Zaki and Ochsner, 2011, p. 175

INTRODUCTION

The aim of part III is not to present an exhaustive overview of neurobiological research and theories concerning autism. Rather, we hope that our relatively brief and highly selective neurobiological summary will allow the reader to have a more immediate grasp of how neurobiological and psychological factors are intertwined in ASD. Perhaps the reader will even be able to experience some of our amazement and excitement that so many independent voices from such diverse backgrounds, including psychoanalysis, seem to be speaking in unison to express a similar conclusion regarding ASD—namely that *ASD can be thought of as a potentially reversible neurodevelopmental disorder with experiential/psychological consequences, for example, the experience of deprivation of growth-promoting parental input, which contribute significantly to the development and maintenance of autistic impairments and suffering* (Mahler, 1968; Greenspan, 1992; Dawson, 2008; Herbert & Weintraub, 2012; Helt et al., 2008; Pelphrey & Carter, 2008; Szalavitz & Perry, 2010; Sherkow, 2005, 2011; Singletary, 2006, 2009). However, because of the relative isolation of these efforts, this confluence of thought has not, to our knowledge, previously been appreciated. In addition, the emotional and psychological impact of such altered neurobiological functioning—the meaning to the young child—in general, has not been emphasized. This chapter will offer a possible framework for understanding the mechanisms through which psychoanalytic treatment and the more general application of psychoanalytic understanding could lead to neuroplastic changes and, thus, be helpful in the treatment of ASD, a neurobiological disorder. We are attempting to bring together multiple perspectives in a new way, one that is mutually enriching for both psychoanalysis and neurobiology and can lead to testable hypotheses and generative, interdisciplinary research. We believe that this path will lead to a deeper and richer understanding of ASD and to the use of psychoanalytic understanding and insights to develop more effective and proven treatments to benefit children with ASD and their families. All in all, this chapter will suggest a neurobiological foundation to support the crucial importance of understanding the child's psychological experience and meaning—what a 10-year-old boy in treatment for Asperger's referred to as "the missing piece" of the autism puzzle. With this background, it would seem natural to include psychoanalytic contributions and dynamic therapy as part of the treatment of ASD.

OVERVIEW OF THE NEUROBIOLOGY OF AUTISM

Autism is an extremely complex, heterogeneous neurodevelopmental disorder involving what is being discovered to be an ever-growing number of genes and multiple biological mechanisms. These factors interfere with brain development and functioning at many levels, leading to the disruption of brain circuits mediating language and behavioral flexibility as well as social cognition and interaction (Abrahams & Geschwind, 2010; Geschwind & Levitt, 2007; DiCicco-Bloom et al., 2006; Amaral et al., 2008). Thus, there are numerous forms of autism with many different neurobiological pathways all converging to shape the individual's experience and to lead to the clinical manifestations of ASD (Zimmerman, 2008; Amaral et al., 2008; DiCicco-Bloom et al., 2006; Herbert & Anderson, 2008; Greenspan & Shanker, 2004; Siegel, 2007).

TENTATIVE WORKING MODEL

In order to place our review of individual neurobiological factors in context, we will begin with a tentative working model that lays the groundwork for a possible conceptualization of this pathological process (Singletary, 2009). A number of neurobiological factors are thought to interact and form a complex nonlinear network, which includes child-parent interactions and the individual's own experiences and meanings, all resulting in the syndrome of ASD (see figure 8.1).

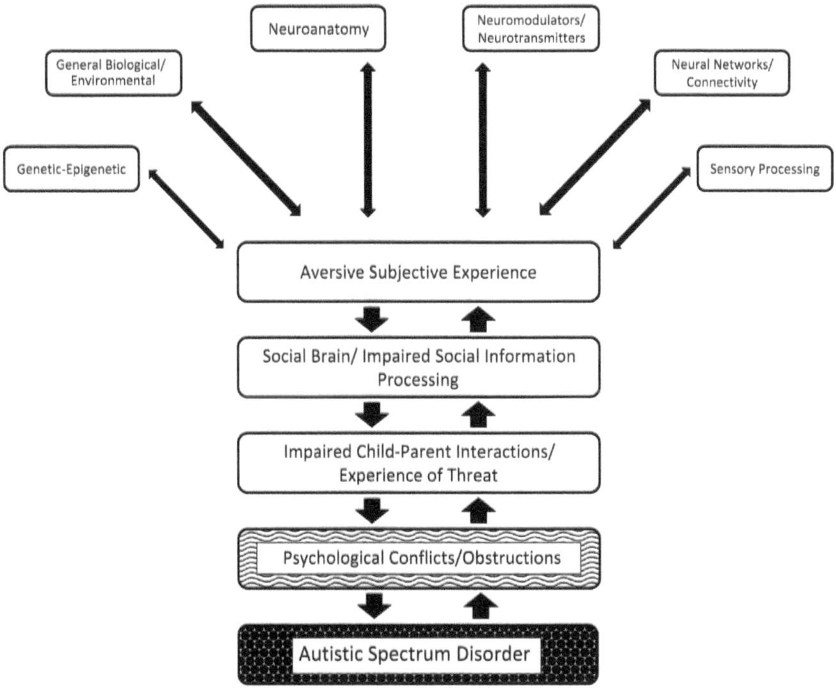

Figure 8.1. The Many Paths to ASD

While, as noted above, ASD is a disorder of great complexity and uncertain etiology, autism has been linked to a number of broad factors including genetic and epigenetic contributions and other general biological factors such as neuroinflammation, immune function, and nutrition, as well as diverse environmental influences such as maternal-fetal interaction, toxins, and infections. In addition, neuroanatomy as well as neuromodulators and neurotransmitters have an impact. At still another level, synaptic function, connectivity, neural networks, and sensory processing play a crucial role. All of these factors interact and converge. This leads to increased aversive subjective experience, for example, overarousal in response to novel, unpredictable stimuli such as social information (Dawson & Lewy, 1989), which, in a bidirectional interaction, disrupts the functioning of the social brain. The subsequent impaired social information processing, cognition, empathic accuracy, and social motivation in combination negatively impact the child's relationships and subjective psychological experience. These neurobiological elements obstruct the infant's experience of comforting relationships with caregivers, thereby impeding the child's feeling a sense of safety and calm well-being. Consider the recent statement by Pelphrey and Carter (2008) concerning social isolation in autism: "In the case of the child with autism, there is no doubt that parents, grandparents, siblings, and educators provide an abundance of love, warmth, and care, but the child does not develop the brain mechanisms that allow him or her to reach out and take hold of this social fabric" (p. 1084).

The related autism literature has concentrated almost exclusively on the critically important consequences of such deprivation at the level of the social brain, highlighting the *developmental, social deficits*, which interfere with adaptive parent-child interaction. With this emphasis, helpful psychosocial treatment has consisted almost entirely of behavioral/developmental interventions which, while most important, are limited because they exclude the child's inner world. In this book we hope to increase awareness that *psychological conflicts* engendered by the infant's experience of neurobiologically driven deprivation and social isolation also play a significant part in obstructing adaptive parent-child interaction. As we are demonstrating, the meanings for the child of such early and ongoing pathological experiences need to be considered. Tronick and Beeghley (2011) underscore the importance of infant meaning-making in developmental outcome. While these meanings are made at a biopsychosocial level and are nonsymbolic, they do shape ongoing parent-child interactions and, when aberrant, can interfere with adaptive engagement with others and contribute to pathological outcomes (Tronick & Beeghley, 2011).

While there may be many emotional and psychological reactions to the neurobiologically based developmental experience of early deprivation, one possible example will serve to illustrate the interplay between emotional and psychological conflicts and the social brain. Deprived of appropriate neurobiological input, the child fails to experience mother's comforting presence and protection, and, instead registers heightened anxiety, stress, and a sense of threat (Mahler, 1968). Even with loving reactions from parents, the child may make inaccurate and pathological meanings of these experiences and conclude that human interactions are not only unrewarding, but also frightening and must be avoided. Thus, the child's efforts to make sense of and cope with the experience of aloneness and danger could lead to a defensive withdrawal from others and to psychological conflicts regarding relationships. For example, the child could feel both a great need for emotional contact with parents and, simultaneously, a dread of such closeness. This heightened anxiety and fear surrounding the world of people and the ensuing social isolation would further hinder accurate social cognition and empathic accuracy and, to an even greater degree, interfere with social motivation and adaptive social interaction. In a vicious circle, the child's self-regulating and protective efforts could further constrain adaptive parent-child interaction. Thus, these interlocking neurobiological and emotional/psychological impairments come together in a final common pathway leading to the various clinical manifestations of the syndrome of ASD, in both its development and maintenance (Singletary, 2009; Sherkow, 2011).

It is crucial to keep in mind that all of these influences are bidirectional. In pathogenesis, numerous vicious circles—both within and among all of these different factors (Herbert & Weintraub, 2012; Singletary, 2009; Sherkow, 2011)—are established and interact in ways that lead to increasing disturbance. For example, neuroinflammation can interfere with neural connectivity and social cognition, which can lead to social withdrawal and increased stress, which, in turn, can increase neuroinflammation (Herbert & Weintraub, 2012).

Another related example will demonstrate the multiple points at which such interactions occur. A factor such as abnormally enlarged white matter which weakens connections between the prefrontal cortex and other regions of the brain and, thereby, impedes integrative functioning (Kana et al., 2008; Herbert et al., 2004; Minshew et al., 2008) may act in combination with increased connectivity within the frontal lobe (Scott-Van Zeeland et al., 2010). Together these can contribute to hypersensitivity to sensory stimulation and social information, which in turn can interfere with emotional regulation as well as social cognition and empathic accuracy and impede both social motivation and interactions. Thus, as described above, such *neurobiological deficits* or obstructions in social interactions at the level of the social brain can lead to *psychological conflicts* which further interfere with and obstruct relationships. Thus, autism is not solely a developmental disorder with social deficits to be dealt with by only behavioral, developmental, and biomedical interventions. Treatment of patients with autistic spectrum disorder must account for both its neurobiological and its experiential dimensions. When considering neuroplasticity, we will present evidence that, with appropriate intervention, an upward spiral can be established and reverse this pathological process. This review of neurobiology and neuroplasticity in autism will provide a foundation for investigating and understanding the mechanisms whereby taking into account the child's internal conflicts can make a substantial contribution to treatment.

GENETIC AND EPIGENETIC MECHANISMS

This brief overview will clearly indicate some of the numerous ways that genetic factors can interfere with the functioning of the social brain and emotional experience through disruptive effects on the functioning of crucial brain regions, neural pathways, and neuromodulators. Such interferences with the workings of the social brain will adversely impact emotional regulation (Mazefsky, Pelphrey, & Dahl, 2012) and parent-child interactions (Dawson, 2008). In addition, Dawson (2008) proposes that the resulting altered interactions between child and parents might lead to epigenetic changes and amplify the influences of autism susceptibility genes.

Despite recent research indicating that the heritability rate for ASD is significantly less than the earlier estimate of greater than 90 percent and that shared environmental factors in the prenatal and early postnatal periods make a significant contribution to the susceptibility to ASD (Hallmayer et al., 2011), there is overwhelming evidence that genetic factors play a pivotal role (DiCicco-Bloom et al., 2006; Amaral et al., 2008). The siblings of autistic individuals are over 20 times more likely to have ASD than the general population, and apparently unaffected siblings have been shown to share with the autistic sibling similar brain responses to certain stimuli, including such psychologically meaningful stimuli as the facial expression of emotion (Spencer, Holt, & Chura, 2011; Belmonte, Gormot, & Baron-Cohen, 2010; Dalton, Nacewicz, Alexander, & Davidson, 2007).

Through a number of mechanisms, genetic factors can interfere with the development and functioning of the brain and can (as in figure 8.1) "disrupt neural systems that process cognition and social behaviors" (Amaral et al., 2008, p. 385). Some genetic abnormalities may disrupt neural processes involving synaptic formation and function (neuroligin/neurexin) and therefore produce widespread interference (Amaral et al., 2008). For example, variants in the autism risk gene CNTNAP2 (a member of the neurexin superfamily) have been found to predispose an individual to autism through modulation of frontal lobe connectivity, that is, increased connectivity within the frontal lobe and decreased connectivity with other parts of the brain (Scott-Van Zeeland et al., 2010). This finding is of obvious importance since the frontal lobe is crucial for a number of higher-order cognitive, social, and communication functions and is implicated in the mirror neuron system (Scott-Van Zeeland et al., 2010) as well as in joint attention (Mundy, 2003). In fact, Geschwind and Levitt (2007, pp. 105–6), propose that such disruptions, that is, "disconnection of dorsolateral prefrontal regions and anterior cingulate cortex from other regions necessary to develop joint attention in early infancy, which is the foundation of language and social behavior, would probably have widespread reverberations during development" and suggest that autism spectrum disorders be considered *disconnection syndromes*.

On the other hand, variants involving other genes which are expressed in neurons having certain features in common, for example, participation in a particular circuit or involving a particular neuromodulator (oxytocin and vasopressin receptors in the hypothalamus and amygdala), will cause more localized or well-defined difficulties (Amaral et al., 2008). For example, despite some recent contradictory evidence (Tansey et al., 2010), both genetic and epigenetic variations in the oxytocin receptor (OXTR) gene have been linked to an increased risk of autism (Gregory et al., 2009; Wu et al., 2005; Jacob et al., 2007; Lerer et al., 2007; Liu et al., 2010). Also, variants in some ASD-associated genes have been linked to the development of brain structures which have consistently been found to be abnormal in ASD, for example, ENGRAILED2, a regulator of cerebellar development (Rossman & Di-Cicco-Bloom, 2008). (The significance of both oxytocin and the cerebellum for social and emotional development will each be discussed below.)

In addition, it is most interesting to discover a mouse model, which connects the behavioral manifestations of ASD to increased anxiety and to an altered relationship to mother as in our model. Researchers have developed a chromosome-engineered mouse model for 15q11-13 duplication, which has been linked to ASD. These mice show impaired social interaction, inflexible behavior, increased distress signals in response to maternal separation as pups, and increased anxiety (Nakatani et al., 2009).

GENERAL BIOLOGICAL/ENVIRONMENTAL FACTORS

The group of general biological/environmental factors thought to play a significant role in either the development or the ongoing manifestations of ASD encompasses an extremely broad and heterogeneous assemblage of influences, for example, neuroinflammation, immune function, nutrition, and toxins. Indeed, in some of these "environmental" factors such as altered patterns of social interaction—considered to be a risk process for the development of ASD—both genetic and epigenetic elements may be at work (Dawson, 2008). For a clear example, we can return to Dawson's model (2008) where genetic risk factors can lead to altered infant-parent interactions (an environmental factor) which, in turn, can magnify the effects of the initial autism susceptibility genes.

As mentioned above, recent evidence for the importance of shared environmental factors among twins with ASD has highlighted the importance of the prenatal and early postnatal environment for autism susceptibility (Hallmayer et al., 2011). These nongenetic risk factors include maternal illnesses during pregnancy, environmental toxins during pregnancy, maternal-fetal immunoreactivity, parental age, low birth weight, and twinning (Hallmayer et al., 2011; Szatmari, 2011).

The risk to children posed by environmental toxins is of particular concern since there is much support for the idea that the developing brain is extremely vulnerable to the impact of toxins (Herbert & Weintraub, 2012). The fact that genetic factors in ASD can heighten the adverse effects triggered by exposures (Pessah & Lein, 2008; Herbert, 2010b; Herbert & Weintraub, 2012) makes the threat due to environmental toxins of even greater concern. Herbert (2005a) has postulated that environmental toxins could contribute to an increased "excitation-inhibition ratio" in ASD and that "the degree of environmental exposure may affect both whether genetic vulnerability turns into disease and how severe this disease becomes" (p. 2).

In light of the role that the experience of threat and heightened anxiety may play in ASD, it is extremely interesting that prenatal stress, including such factors as prenatal exposure to hurricanes and tropical storms, has been associated with an increased risk of ASD (Kinney et al., 2008a; Kinney et al., 2008b). (This may be particularly important because of its possible effects on the locus coeruleus-noradrenergic system to be discussed later.)

NEUROANATOMY

As in other areas in ASD, neuroanatomical considerations are certainly not clear-cut and straightforward. In their overview, Amaral et al. (2008) emphasize that ASD does not involve a single region of the brain and that there may be phenotypic variations in brain pathology. The amygdala, the fusiform face area (as it relates to the amygdala), and the cerebellum are of particular importance.

First, the amygdala is involved in the fear circuits of the brain including the evaluation of stimuli for threat and the detection of danger, emotional memory, fear conditioning, fear extinction (critical to the possibility of change), and the evaluation of facial expressions (LeDoux, 2000). In addition, the amygdala is linked to the emotional processing of sensory information and plays a role in moderating social interactions (Meaney et al., 2008; Amaral et al., 2008). The amygdala also projects to the locus coeruleus-noradrenergic system (LeDoux, 2000). The recent model of ASD (Mehler & Purpura, 2009) (to be discussed in section 2), which emphasizes the role of the locus coeruleus-noradrenergic system, makes this amygdalar connection of even greater significance.

While earlier research led to an "amygdala theory of autism" which postulated a hypoactive amygdala (Baron-Cohen et al., 2000), more recent research supports a model of amygdala hyperactivity (Dalton et al., 2005; Dalton et al., 2006; Nacewicz et al., 2006). When processing faces, subjects with autism were found to have hypoactivation in the fusiform gyrus and increased activation in the amygdala. This finding was considered to suggest a heightened emotional response to gaze fixation and a hypersensitivity to social stimuli in autism (Dalton et al., 2005). Such disruptions in processing of social and emotional stimuli could lead to the problems in social behavior associated with ASD (Rossman & DiCicco-Bloom, 2008). Recently, Kleinhans et al. (2009) found that, in response to socially relevant stimuli, adults with ASD showed reduced neural habituation in the amygdala and concluded that the social deficits observed in ASD may be related to sustained amygdala arousal. Interestingly, in healthy adults individual attachment style has been found to modulate amygdala and striatum activation to facial expressions such "that secure attachment may correspond to a combination of low anxiety and low avoidance" (Vrtička et al., 2008, p.7). This provides a clear example of how internal relationships affect the activity of the brain—of how psychological factors affect neurobiological functioning.

The cerebellum is another brain region thought to play a significant role in social processing (Cozolino, 2006) and to be of importance in ASD. Both neuroanatomically and functionally, the cerebellum (Courchesne, Webb, & Schurmann, 2011) has been consistently found to be abnormal in ASD patients. In fact, the gene ENGRAILED2, which regulates cerebellar development, has been considered to be an ASD-susceptibility gene (Rossman & DiCicco-Bloom, 2008). Also, the cerebellum has been found to be involved in higher order functions of particular importance in ASD including attention regulation and speech (Rossman & DiCicco-Bloom, 2008). Interestingly, Cozolino (2006) considers the cerebellum to be a "hub of social processing" and focuses primarily on the cerebellum in his consideration of the social difficulties found in autism. In addition to the cerebellum's role in the coordination of motor function and in balance and equilibrium, he suggests that the cerebellum may be important in the timing and modulation of language and affective regulation. According to Cozolino (2006, p. 288), cerebellar damage "appears to disrupt many of the very functions that serve as the basis for vital interpersonal attunement" and to interfere with the development of empathy and interpersonal relationships. Obviously, this suggests one pathway whereby impaired neurobiological functioning could contribute to a pathological experience of isolation and danger and, thus, to the ultimate development of the ASD syndrome.

NEUROMODULATORS AND NEUROTRANSMITTERS

A number of neurotransmitters and neuromodulators including oxytocin, glutamate, dopamine, norepinephrine, serotonin, endogenous opiods, and acetylcholine have been implicated in ASD. However, we will limit our discussion to oxytocin and glutamate, both of which are likely to be involved in crucial ways.

Oxytocin

Based on their roles in forming social attachments in nonhuman mammals, the neuromodulators, oxytocin and vasopressin, have long been considered to be of likely significance in ASD (Insel, 1997). Since at least 1997, a growing body of evidence has demonstrated oxytocin's role in facilitating human connectedness and interactions. In healthy human subjects oxytocin has been shown to improve the ability to understand the mental state of others from subtle social cues (Domes et al., 2007a), reduce amygdala responses to angry, fearful, and happy facial expressions (Domes et al., 2007b), increase focus on the eye region of human faces (Guastella et al., 2008), and increase trust (Kosfeld et al., 2005). Oxytocin has also been shown to play a somewhat complex role in attachment representations. After the administration of intranasal oxytocin less anxiously attached individuals were found to have more positive recollections of maternal care and closeness in contrast to more anxiously attached individuals who had more negative recollections (Bartz et al., 2010b). In addition, oxytocin has been shown to improve empathic accuracy but only in those who are less socially proficient (Bartz et al., 2010a). Moreover, in healthy subjects, oxytocin receptor gene variation is linked to increased stress reactivity and decreased empathy (Rodrigues et al., 2009).

At this point there is considerable interest in research directly exploring the connection between oxytocin and ASD. As noted above, variations in the oxytocin receptor (OXTR) gene have been linked to an increased risk of autism (Gregory et al., 2009; Wu et al., 2005; Jacob et al., 2007; Lerer et al., 2007; Liu et al., 2010). Another line of evidence is related to clinical trials investigating the effects of IV or intranasal oxytocin in individuals with ASD (Insel, 2010). These initial trials have been suggestive showing reduced repetitive behaviors (Hollander et al., 2003), increased recognition of social information (Hollander et al., 2007), improved recognition of emotion in others (Guastella et al., 2010), and increased social approach and comprehension (Andari et al., 2010) in response to the administration of oxytocin.

Glutamate

Excessive glutamate, the primary excitatory neurotransmitter, leads to a general overreactivity to sensory input (Herbert & Weintraub, 2012). Glutamate seems to play a major role driving excitotoxicity, a pathological process in which excessive levels or activity of glutamate and other excitotoxins damage or kill neurons. Also, an imbalance between excitation and inhibition related to glutamatergic dysregulation has been proposed to modulate numerous risk factors in ASD (Evers & Hollander, 2008) and may play a critical role in causing autism (Herbert & Weintraub, 2012).

NEURAL NETWORKS, CONNECTIVITY, AND PROCESSING

The broad array of factors—ranging from the microscopic to the psychological—involved in our consideration of neural networks, connectivity, and processing are definitely of major importance in the development, maintenance, and treatment of ASD. In pioneering work relating findings in neuroanatomy to processing difficulties in ASD, Herbert et al. (2004) found that the postnatal increase in brain volume (which later normalizes) in autism is caused primarily by white matter enlargement in all lobes, but most strikingly in the prefrontal cortex. They proposed that this abnormal white matter may contribute to pervasive processing deficits. In addition, Herbert (2005b) suggested that chronic, but potentially reversible pathological processes, for example, neuroinflammation, oxidative stress, and excitotoxicity, could generate these disturbances of connectivity and that a widespread "impairment in connectivity or brain integration could underlie the autism behavioral phenotype" (p. 435). Herbert (2005b) added that more complex processes such as subtle language and social interaction and the capacity for behavioral flexibility would be more impaired.

Over many years, Minshew et al. (2008) have developed a highly useful model, the "complex information processing-disconnectivity-neuronal organization model of autism." While there are differences, Minshew and colleagues note certain similarities to other conceptualizations such as the "developmental disconnection syndrome" (Geschwind & Levitt, 2007) mentioned earlier. The model presented by Minshew et al. (2008) includes cortical connection disturbances that, in high functioning ASD, primarily involve increased local frontal connectivity and lessened connectivity among neural systems. This leads to impaired complex information processing including disturbances in processing social information that are connected to the social impairments seen in ASD. For example, Kana et al. (2008) found a functional underconnectivity between frontal and posterior regions in the brain during the attribution of mental states in adults with autism. In addition, Bachevalier and Loveland (2006) have presented evidence that difficulties in self-regulation of social-emotional behavior in ASD are related to dysfunction of the orbitofrontal-amygdala circuit in the brain. Finally, a recent fMRI study involving high-functioning adolescents with ASD compared to normal adolescents found significant decreases in connectivity among three regions of the social brain in those with ASD (Gotts et al., 2012). Specifically, the affective processing limbic region was less connected with the brain regions more involved in the language/communication aspects of social behavior and the brain regions supporting socially relevant sensorimotor processes, that is, the visual perception of "socially relevant form and action" (Gotts et al., 2012, p. 11). Adolescents with ASD who showed the greatest decreases in connectivity among the social brain regions were found to have more severe social symptoms (Gotts et al., 2012). The "thinking brain" does indeed seem to be disconnected from the "feeling brain" (Sherkow, 2007).

In focusing on the autistic mind, Bryson (2005) links information processing to emotion and thought. She concludes that in autism, the mind is hypersensitive to sensory stimulation and vulnerable to sensory overload and adapts to this overarousal by narrowing the focus of attention. This hypersensitivity extends to the emotions, which can be experienced as overwhelming and—because of this heightened intensity and difficulties in reflecting on thoughts and experiences—are poorly modulated by thought. Thus, emotionally significant events lead to narrowed attention and a heightened tendency to engage in repetitive (self-regulating) behaviors. She adds that, "under such circumstances, positive emotion can readily be experienced as aversive" (p. 41). *We feel that this observation is of utmost importance in understanding the experience and behavior of individuals with ASD, which can seem so paradoxical, for example, pleasurable interactions are often followed by disruptions.*

In summary, autism is widely considered to involve increased local connectivity within brain regions and decreased connectivity among more distant brain regions leading to problems in processing tasks requiring "large, highly integrated brain networks such as language and social-emotional functions" (Williams, 2008, p. 14). This conclusion recently received support in a study (Wolff et al., 2012) that found evidence of aberrant development in white matter fiber tracts from 6 to 24 months in infants with autism. These results were seen to suggest that differences in white matter pathways could precede the manifestations of ASD symptoms (Wolff et al., 2012). With this early deviation in the development of white matter fiber tracts in mind, recent research demonstrating that behavioral/cognitive intervention can bring about a positive change in cortical connectivity through alteration of white matter tracts in children (Keller & Just, 2009) has major implications for prevention and early intervention (Dawson, 2012).

These recent developments regarding the importance of cortical connectivity and white matter fiber tracts in ASD along with the possibility of positively affecting these connections through alteration of white matter tracts as a result of behavioral intervention certainly highlights the possibility that psychoanalytic treatment, intervening at a cognitive level, can bring about beneficial neuroplastic changes in children with ASD.

NEUROPLASTICITY

A 2009 neuroscience workshop sponsored by the National Institutes of Health Blueprint for Neuroscience Research led to the definition of neuroplasticity as "the ability of the nervous system to respond to intrinsic or extrinsic stimuli by reorganizing its structure, function and connections" (Cramer et al., 2011, p. 1592). It is crucial to recognize that *intrinsic stimuli*, for example, thoughts, have the capacity to alter brain structure (including connectivity) and function. The authors (Cramer et al., 2011) consider cognitive training to be analogous to physical therapy involving the non-motor brain. Cramer et al. (2011, p. 1600) conclude that, "Evidence suggests that, as individuals learn to modify their cognitive representations and behavioral responses to distressing stimuli, widespread changes occur in frontal cognitive control systems and in limbic system activation." In reaching this conclusion, they cite two PET studies (Goldapple et al., 2004; Kennedy et al.,

2007) involving the effects of CBT in depression and one fMRI study (Farb et al., 2010) examining the effects of mindfulness training on the neural expression of sadness. This lends further support to our proposal that psychoanalytic treatment can have a beneficial effect in the treatment of ASD.

Over 30 years ago, Eric Kandel raised the possibility that psychotherapy works through producing neuroplastic changes (1979). A few years later, he (Kandel, 1983) emphasized that experience modifies the function of the brain through alteration of the strength of synapses and regulating the expression of genes. Most importantly, for our consideration of neuroplasticity in the treatment of ASD, Kandel (1983) suggested that psychotherapy could involve the unlearning of anxiety and lead to long-term structural and functional changes in the brain resulting from altered genetic expression. Since then, neuroplasticity, the capacity of neurons to change in structure and alter their connections to each other as the brain adapts to experience over time (Cozolino, 2010), has been the subject of considerable neurobiological research. Also, the relationship between neuroplasticity, psychotherapy, and psychoanalysis has become more widely appreciated (Cozolino, 2002, 2010; Doidge, 2007).

NEUROPLASTICITY IN ASD

However, some recent developments were necessary in order to bring neuroplasticity into the foreground in the study of autism. Of paramount importance have been neurobiological models of ASD which emphasize dynamic and reversible impairments of brain function instead of fixed, genetic brain defects (Herbert, 2005a, 2005b; Herbert & Anderson, 2008; Dawson, 2008). In addition, a recent prospective study (Curran et al., 2007) found that children with ASD showed improvements in behavior with decreases in stereotypy, irritability, and hyperactivity as well as improved speech both during and briefly after significant febrile episodes. In my own clinical experience, some parents have reported dramatic changes in their children with ASD during fevers. In stark contrast to their usual behavior, during febrile episodes, some children are able to engage in lengthy emotionally meaningful conversations. For example, most uncharacteristically, one 7-year-old boy talked to his mother about how he could really see how much his father loved him because his dad had taken such good care of him in the middle of the night when he was vomiting.

Curran et al. (2007) offered possible explanations for this rapid but short-lived change including modification of neuronal and synaptic function and involvement of the HPA axis with resultant modifications in neurotransmitters. This suggests that—at least in some children with ASD—the malfunctioning neural circuits are intact but obstructed by some unknown, but potentially reversible, factor(s). Subsequently there has been significant interest in understanding the neurobiological mechanisms underlying this improvement (Fischbach, 2010; Moorman, 2010; Mehler & Purpura, 2009) with particular focus on the hypothalamus and its effect on both the release of oxytocin and vasopressin as well as on the locus coeruleus-noradrenergic system (Mehler & Purpura, 2009; Fischbach, 2010; Moorman, 2010). It is interesting to note that Panksepp (Panksepp, 1998; Panksepp, Nelson, & Bekkedal, 1997), who relates ASD to dysfunction of the separation-distress system, also connects the separation-distress and the social comfort systems with thermoregulation, oxytocin, and the hypothalamus such that on a "neurosymbolic" level the perception of social loss is associated with feeling cold and warmth with reunion.

In addition to febrile illness, other conditions lead to sudden but transient improvement in ASD. For example, Herbert and Weintraub (2012) note that treatment with steroids or antibiotics for conditions such as asthma can lead to rapid improvement in social interaction and communication in children with autism which vanishes when these medications are discontinued.

Herbert and Weintraub (2012) also highlight the work of Beversdorf (Narayanan et al., 2010) demonstrating rapid, transient increases in functional connectivity between brain regions in ASD following the administration of propranolol. They (Herbert & Weintraub, 2012) underscore propranolol's use in the treatment of anxiety and suggest a role for psychological stress in creating connectivity problems in ASD. Furthermore, Beversdorf (Narayanan et al., 2010) postulates that propranolol could act through modulation of the noradrenergic system and notes the potential connection between their findings and the Mehler and Purpura (2009) hypothesis concerning the role of the locus coeruleus-noradrenergic system in ASD. (We will discuss this hypothesis in section 2.)

Table 8.1. Factors Promoting Positive Change in ASD

• Fever • Steroids • Antibiotics • Propanolol • Stress and Anxiety Reduction	• Normalizing Environmental Input (Social and Emotional Engagement)	• Intensive Practice and Effort

Of great clinical significance, in a recent review Helt et al. (2008) estimate that between 3 and 25 percent of children with autism recover, that is, lose the diagnosis of ASD, as well as become able to function in the normal range socially, cognitively, and adaptively. This group then provides a detailed consideration of neuroplasticity and possible mechanisms for recovery. They conclude that controlled studies involving the use of behavioral techniques which report the most recovery are intensive (> 20 hours per week) and involve the parents. They also assert that "competent behavioral therapy requires a highly affective, emotionally positive set of interactions that promote the reward value of social interactions and more or less continuous social engagement, especially in very young children" (Helt et al., 2008, p. 350). In addition, child characteristics predicting recovery included higher intelligence, imitation, receptive language, the milder diagnosis of Asperger's Syndrome or PDD-NOS rather than AD, along with earlier age of diagnosis and treatment. Before considering their formulations regarding neuroplasticity in the pathogenesis and recovery from ASD, we will briefly consider the concept of neuroplasticity itself.

NEUROPLASTICITY IN GENERAL

In neurobiology, as noted above, one of the major recent developments has been the dramatic rise in our understanding of the brain's capacity to change—neuroplasticity. According to Hebb's Law, "neurons that fire together wire together" (Doidge, 2007, p. 223; Hebb, 1949). Thus, the brain operates in a "use it or lose it" fashion referred to as "use-dependent plasticity" (Cozzolino, 2010, p. 325). Considering brain development to be self-organizing and using a dynamic systems theory model, Lewis (2005) describes cortical developmental change as a reorganization of synaptic connections between neurons, which change and stabilize based on neuronal activity. Stabilization in the cortex and limbic system occurs because of synaptic sculpting so that these synaptic structural changes become self-perpetuating (Lewis, 2005). The mechanism of "cascading constraints," such that early developmental structures limit characteristics of structures evolving later, contributes to the developmental trajectory of an individual (Lewis, 2005). Thus, alongside of the potential for progressive development of the brain in an optimal fashion, there exists the possibility for maladaptive plasticity or pathological brain organization (Helt et al., 2008). Herbert and Weintraub (2012) repeatedly call attention to the operation of such vicious circles at multiple points and levels in the pathological processes leading to autistic impairments.

Taub (Doidge, 2007; Begley, 2007; Taub, 2008; Taub et al., 2004) has described a similar mechanism which may contribute to progressive pathological organization in the brain—"learned nonuse"—a primarily behavioral phenomenon, which contributes to actual brain atrophy, a related neural mechanism. In this case, individuals sustaining cerebral insults, such as cerebral palsy or stroke, may—in a vicious circle—come to use the more-affected limb less because of greater residual difficulty. However, such disuse can be overcome and the brain atrophy reversed by treatment involving restricted use of the less-affected limb and intensive training of the more-affected limb (Doidge, 2007; Begley, 2007; Taub et al., 2004; Taub, 2008). Both restricted use of the stronger limb and intensively training the weaker limb are central aspects of Constraint-Induced Movement therapy. While originally developed for treatment of stroke and traumatic brain injuries in adults, this innovative treatment was recently successfully adapted to treat infants as young as 7 months and older children with cerebral palsy (Taub et al., 2004). Thus, properly applied, the brain's capacity for neuroplasticity can be used to reverse some pathological processes and effectively treat serious neurobiologically based disorders.

The analogy between Taub's (Taub et al., 2004) highly effective intervention for infants with CP and Dawson's (2008) proposal that early intervention can possibly prevent ASD must be underscored. Perhaps the treatment of infants with cerebral palsy (Taub et al., 2004), a neurodevelopmental disorder, could best be considered an example of secondary prevention through intensive early intervention. Obviously, all of these related mechanisms are of considerable interest and have important implications for the pathogenesis, treatment of, and possible recovery from ASD (Helt et al., 2008).

Before turning to a consideration of neuroplasticity and therapeutic intervention in ASD, we will briefly consider some other general aspects of neuroplasticity. First, neuroplasticity requires motivation, attention, and effort (Begley, 2007; Doidge, 2007; Taub, 2008). Second, there is evidence of both rapid and slower—but more permanent—changes, with the rapid changes involving strengthening of existing synaptic connections and the slower changes reflecting the growth of new structures, for example, new neuronal connections (Doidge, 2007; Pascual-Leone et al., 1998). Finally, there is considerable evidence that, although more limited than in early childhood, neuroplasticity continues well into adulthood, if not over the entire lifespan (Begley, 2007; Doidge, 2007).

NEUROPLASTICITY AND THERAPEUTIC INTERVENTION IN ASD

The previously mentioned Keller and Just (2009) study is an important example of neuroplasticity extending beyond early childhood. This neuroimaging study found that 100 hours of intensive remedial reading instruction provided to 8- to 12-year-old children who were poor readers brought about a positive change in cortical connectivity as well as improvement in reading ability. The neuroimaging data revealed changes in white matter thought to suggest increased myelination. This raises the possibility for effective intervention which alters the function and basic structure of the brain much beyond early childhood for individuals with ASD. In fact, Bergman (2012) has found considerable improvement in a patient with ASD through middle age.

In general, effective psychotherapy may be considered to represent a type of enriched environment that stimulates or enhances adaptive neuroplasticity (Cozolino, 2010) through neural network growth and integration, epigenetic mechanisms (Kandel, 1983), moderating levels of stress or states of arousal, affect regulation, repairing attachment schemas, and the creation of a powerful healing relationship or, in cognitive neuroscience terms, the placebo effect which is seen to be a social phenomenon which has powerful neurobiological effects, especially on the regulation of emotion (Cozolino, 2010; Ochsner et al., 2004).

Before turning to our specific consideration of ASD treatment and neuroplasticity, we will restate our basic hypothesis about the pathogenic process in ASD and add our model of the process of change and positive neuroplasticity in the therapy of ASD. Again, ASD is a neurobiological disorder that leads to increased aversive subjective experience and disrupts the functioning of the social brain—including social cognition and motivation. In turn, this results in both impaired relationships and psychological conflicts regarding emotional connections. These psychological consequences further obstruct growth-promoting child-parent interactions and negatively impact subsequent brain development (see figure 8.2).

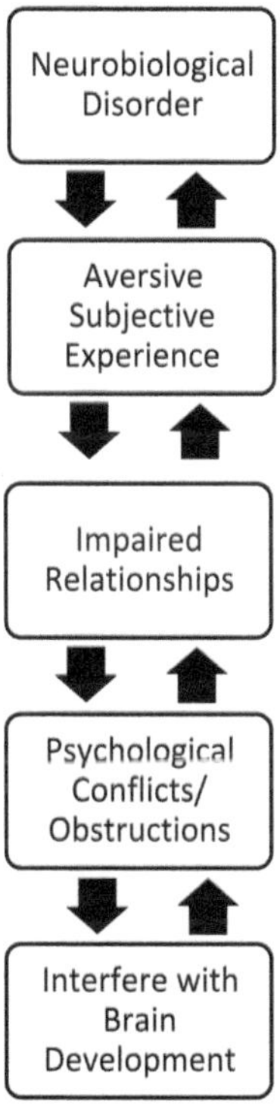

Figure 8.2. Negative Neuroplasticity in ASD

However, in addition to such vicious circles, Lewis' mechanism of cascading constraints (Lewis, 2005) offers the possibility for positive neuroplasticity and establishment of progressive upward spirals in relationships and brain development. In our model we focus on what has been a missing element in neurobiological considerations of ASD and its behavioral/developmental treatment—the child's subjective experience, its meaning, and the resultant psychological conflicts (see figure 8.3).

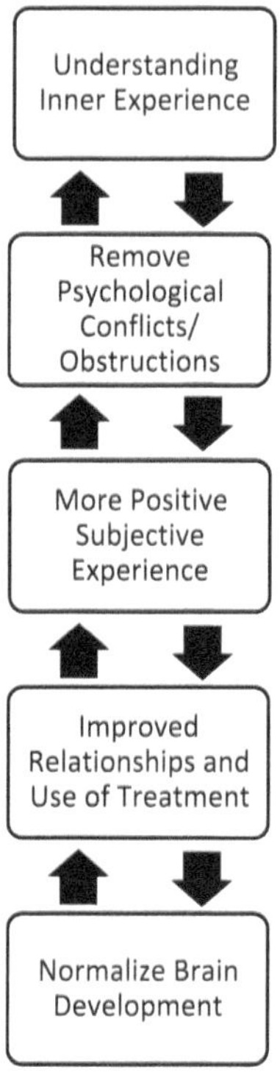
Understanding Inner Experience
Remove Psychological Conflicts/ Obstructions
More Positive Subjective Experience
Improved Relationships and Use of Treatment
Normalize Brain Development

Figure 8.3. Positive Neuroplasticity in ASD

In his recent book, *Be Different* (2011), John Elder Robison, who refers to himself as an Aspergerian, describes having shown his therapist a documentary about a 16-year-old boy with Asperger's in which Robison had identified the boy's fear as he walked the school halls "constantly. . . . Looking for threats. . . . Like a lone deer in a forest filled with wolves. . . . I knew exactly how he felt. . . . Alone, scared . . . no one around him understood him" (p. 3). Robison contrasted his reading of the boy's behavior with that of his therapist's superficial response, seeing only "furtive eye movements . . . [that are] common in people with autism. It doesn't mean anything" (pp. 3–4). Robison felt as if he had "been punched in the gut. . . . Every expression and gesture means something. It's sometimes hard to figure out what the meaning is, but it always exists. . . ." (p. 4). Understanding meanings can make a most substantial contribution to treatment.

Now, turning to the specific consideration of ASD treatment, recovery, and potential mechanisms of change and neuroplasticity, Helt et al. (2008) make the most interesting suggestion that perhaps ASD could be considered to be a syndrome of early deprivation based upon neurobiological, and not environmental, factors. However, they note that despite obvious similarities that there are certainly differences between ASD and environmental deprivation and that environmental deprivation alone does not lead to the full ASD syndrome. In addition, they note other arguments against this formulation. Nevertheless, they point out that three of their mechanisms—"normalizing input through forcing of attention," "promoting reinforcement value of social stimuli," and "early intervention provides an 'enriched environment'"—are all related to normalizing environmental input. In fact, virtually all of their mechanisms are compatible with the suggestion that ASD could be usefully thought of as a syndrome of neurobiologically based environmental deprivation. Therefore, it is quite possible that (1) early neurobiological factors in the infant interfere with necessary environmental input from caregivers which then plays a major role in the development of ASD (Dawson, 2008) and that (2) reversing this process is the cornerstone of ASD treatment (Dawson, 2008). Helt et al. (2008) also point out that their suggestions regarding mechanisms of change are all compatible with Dawson's (2008) model which we will consider in more detail in the following chapter.

Helt et al. (2008) provide a detailed discussion of each of these mechanisms:

1. Normalizing input through forcing of attention

   One possibility is that the forcing of attention to social stimuli would help overcome a deficit in attention and/or social motivation that is due to some factor(s) such as overwhelming arousal (Kinsbourne, 1987), sensory overload, or other aversive reaction to social engagement and interrupt a growth-disturbing process of environmental deprivation (Helt et al., 2008) or the "risk process" of altered interaction with the environment (Dawson, 2008).
2. Promoting reinforcement value of social stimuli

   Through helping the child have a positive emotional reaction to people, this mechanism would presumably enable the child to overcome some underlying difficulty in the motivational and emotional systems promoting social interaction (Helt et al., 2008; Dawson, 2008).
3. Early intervention provides an "enriched environment"

   As mentioned above, it is possible that the environment experienced by the ASD child is one of functional deprivation due to neurobiological processes (Helt et al., 2008). Thus, as suggested by Dawson (2008), one mechanism driving successful early intervention may be the creation of an enriched environment for the child (Helt et al., 2008).

4. Early intervention provides mass trialing/practice

This mechanism underscores the crucial importance of *repetitive* exposure and practice in ASD treatment. Since, as noted above, one of the primary factors in effective early intervention is intensity, Helt et al. (2008) raise the possibility of a similarity to Taub et al.'s (2004) Constraint-Induced Movement therapy in which intensive practice is needed to promote neural development by forcing use of a malfunctioning neural system. In addition, Helt et al. (2008) add that effective treatment may need to ensure the child's effort and attention.

5. Compensatory input

Here, Helt et al. (2008) raise the possibility of reversible damage to neural systems subserving key functions, for example, face processing or language. Recovery would depend upon helping the child learn certain pivotal skills through alternate strategies which, rather than facilitating recovery in malfunctioning systems of the brain, would rely upon recruiting new compensatory areas of the brain not generally used for such processes. Taub (Taub et al., 2004; Taub, 2008) found evidence for such cortical reorganization in Constraint-Induced Movement therapy.

6. Effective intervention suppresses interfering behaviors

This mechanism focuses on suppressing behaviors that interfere with connection to others and result in the experience of environmental deprivation, especially repetitive or self-stimulatory behavior (Lewis et al., 2007; Bodfish, 2011). Helt et al. (2008) discuss some hypotheses regarding the functions of repetitive behavior including arousal-reduction (Kinsbourne, 1987) and avoiding sensory overload and stress. Helt et al. (2008) raise the possibility that in ASD, "Many deviant behaviors" could be considered to be "attempts at compensation" (p. 358). *In line with our thinking, Helt et al. (2008) conclude that in treatment it would likely be productive to understand the individual purposes of such behaviors.*

7. Successful early intervention reduces stress and stabilizes arousal

This is related to Kinsbourne's (1987) proposal that social interactions are avoided in ASD because they are unpredictable and lead to overarousal, while attention to objects and routines are more predictable and less arousing (Helt et al., 2008). Helt et al. (2008) raise the most interesting and important possibility that as the ASD child "grows, rather than turning to a nurturing social environment for soothing, he/she may learn to self-regulate by engaging in repetitive, self-stimulatory behaviors, thus making him/her increasingly less available to the outside world at the risk of being overwhelmed" (p. 358; Lewis, et al., 2007).

Furthermore, Helt et al. (2008) call attention to the fact that chronic stress can lead to brain damage during development and could also interfere with the child's using neural systems which are initially intact and note that this would lead to the hypothesis that signs of autonomic arousal or dysfunction should be found in early life. *They conclude that "normalizing the child's arousal levels" could be "the critical mechanism" underlying effective treatment* (Helt et al., 2008, p. 358).

8. Boosting recovery via biomedical treatment

   Helt et al. (2008) note that while biomedical interventions alone do not lead to recovery, they may enhance the effectiveness of behavioral treatment. However, in the future, biomedical interventions may help increase the possibility for recovery by reducing the severity of pathological biological processes, for example, neuroinflammation, which may lead to a heightened response to stress and overwhelming arousal which would then obstruct basic processes such as social motivation (Helt et al., 2008).

The proposed mechanisms of change can be grouped into three major areas—normalizing environmental input (social and emotional engagement), stress and anxiety reduction, and intensive practice and effort (see table 8.1). All of these factors are compatible with psychoanalytic intervention. Such treatment can help normalize environmental input in a several ways. With the younger child, direct involvement with parents in dyadic treatment and helping the parents actively engage their child are crucial (Greenspan & Wieder, 2006). This principle of active engagement (Settlage, 1992) also plays a critical role in child-therapist interaction. In addition, talking and playing about the child's inner world can be extremely helpful in normalizing the child-parent relationship. For example, helping the child face and adequately cope with fears of connectedness, change, and loss can be immensely beneficial in promoting adaptive engagement with others. Such changes can help to reduce stress and anxiety which, in a virtuous circle, leads, not only to more adaptive interactions with parents and other caregivers, but also to positive neurobiological changes, such as decreased neuroinflammation (Herbert & Weintraub, 2012) and improved immune function (Herbert & Weintraub, 2012). The intensive nature of psychoanalytic treatment is critical in facilitating and continuing such major progress.

Chapter Nine

Models of ASD

A Remarkable Confluence

William M. Singletary, MD

> Each [research] started from a different point and, using different approaches, yields findings which are mutually explanatory. I have first spoken of such convergences in a communication on "Experimental Design" (1950b), and stated that in psychoanalysis such a convergence can occupy the place which validation has in experimental psychology.
>
> —Spitz, 1955, p. 215 in Tustin, 1990, p. 77

INTRODUCTION

As we attempt, in this section, to bring to light how researchers from diverse backgrounds seem to be independently reaching similar conclusions regarding the role of early life stress and deprivation in ASD, it seems most fitting that we begin with a quote from Renée Spitz (1955). A psychoanalytic pioneer, in his groundbreaking research Spitz unearthed the striking physical as well as psychological effects of early deprivation (Spitz, 1945). It is even more appropriate that Frances Tustin, a psychoanalytic pioneer in the treatment of autism, used this quote to introduce a chapter in which she asserted that "autistic reactions are at the interface of neurophysiology and psychodynamic psychology" (Tustin, 1990, p. 92) and are related to defensive reactions to extreme early stress. Tustin concluded that "psychotherapists need to have studied such phenomena so that autistic children may be rescued from their encapsulated isolation" (Tustin, 1990, p. 95).

Despite the extreme heterogeneity in autism recently emphasized by Waterhouse (2008, 2013), elucidating an underlying, but generally unrecognized and potentially unifying model of ASD could help promote collaboration.

Such cooperation and synergy could lead to meaningful research and innovative treatment approaches. While there is no one cause of autism and no one autism phenotype, it is quite striking that a number of relatively independent models of ASD seem to be reaching similar conclusions. As we noted in chapter 8, a consensus seems to be emerging that for a substantial number of children on the autism spectrum, *ASD can be considered to be a potentially reversible neurodevelopmental disorder with experiential/psychological consequences, such as early deprivation of growth-promoting parental input, which contribute significantly to the development and maintenance of autistic impairments and suffering* (Mahler, 1968; Greenspan, 1992; Dawson, 2008; Herbert & Weintraub, 2012; Helt et al., 2008; Pelphrey & Carter, 2008; Szalavitz & Perry, 2010; Sherkow, 2005, 2011; Singletary, 2006, 2009). However, this consensus remains somewhat hidden until one considers some recent models of ASD through the lens of the experience of stress in early life.

Finding that the early experience of stress is a source of underlying unity in these models is especially intriguing in light of Thompson and Levitt's (2010) recent proposal that neurobiologically derived stress during early development may underlie neurodevelopmentally based psychiatric disorders. In addition, given the prominent role attributed to the neurobiologically derived disruption of infant-parent interactions and the ensuing experience of early deprivation in the models of ASD under consideration here, it is extremely pertinent that Loman and Gunnar (2010) focus on deprivation and disruptions in parental care as particularly powerful sources of early life stress. Their underscoring the possibility that appropriate intervention could contribute to recovery from early life stress (Loman & Gunnar, 2010) is in accord with considering ASD to be a potentially reversible disorder related to the experience of early deprivation.

Moreover, the work of both McEwen (McEwen & Lasley, 2002; McEwen & Wingfield, 2003) and Sapolsky (1998, 2010), which focuses on the crucial intertwining of the biological and psychological aspects of stress, provides a solid foundation for a model of ASD involving the interplay of biological and psychological factors. Both highlight that thoughts and emotions alone can be primary triggers for the stress response in humans. Biology and psychology then interact to either exacerbate or ameliorate the pathological effects of chronic stress. McEwen (2002) uses the term *allostasis* rather than *homeostasis* in order to emphasize that allostatic systems help provide stability for the body by being able to change themselves in order to adapt or cope with changes in the environment. Allostatic load refers to the pathological process which causes damage when the protective allostatic response functions improperly, for example, when it inappropriately, repeatedly, or chronically mobilizes the body's stress response system. McEwen asserts that "the revelation that the brain could be the target as well as the initiator of the stress response opened the door to understanding many of the problems and illnesses associated with allostatic load" (McEwen & Lasley, 2002, p. 54). The following model illustrates the effects of early life stress and allostatic load on the neurobiological factors central to autism and focuses on the brain in ASD as the target of psychological stress.

Before turning to a detailed consideration of other models, we will begin with an elaboration of the tentative working model depicted in chapter 8 (see figure 8.1). In that diagram the path represented begins with neurobiological factors which lead to environmental deprivation, the experience of threat and psychological conflicts, which results in the impairments found in ASD. This aspect of the pathological process proceeds from the biological to the psychological and ultimately to autistic symptoms.

The path to be described below is essentially an inverse of the process portrayed in chapter 8. In the new diagram the influence of psychological stress upon the brain is foregrounded, thereby emphasizing the vicious cycle at work. This aspect of the pathological process begins with the symptoms of ASD which lead to additional impairment of child-parent interactions and the experience of environmental deprivation which, in turn, causes chronic early life stress and allostatic load, which further interferes with neurobiological functioning in the areas critical to autism (see figure 9.1).

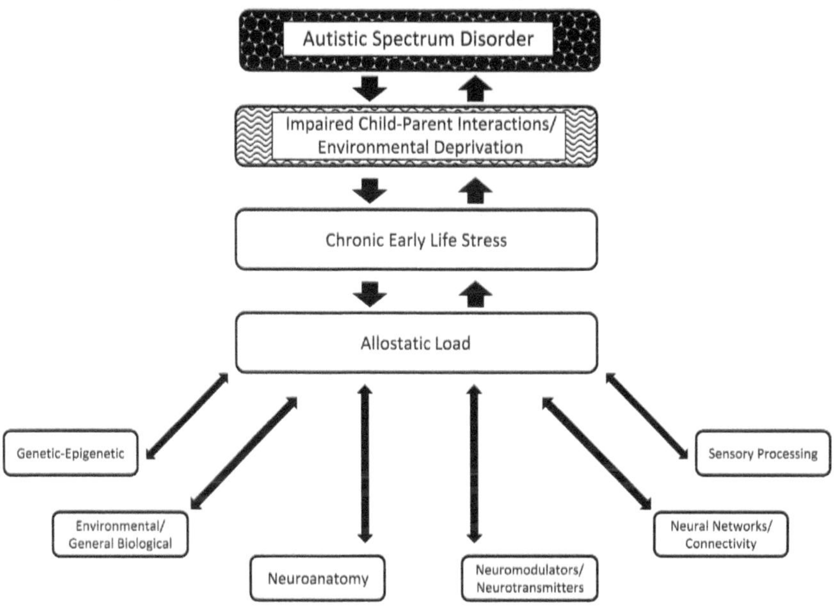

Figure 9.1. Neurobiological Consequences of Environmental Deprivation in ASD

Following is a brief consideration of the various ways in which chronic early life stress impacts the functioning of the brain in the crucial areas noted above:

Genetic/Epigenetic Factors

- Chronic early life stress has been found to lead to long-lasting epigenetic alterations which negatively impact the stress response system and development and, in addition, increase the risk for a number of psychiatric and physical disorders (National Scientific Council on the Developing Child, 2010).

Environmental/General Biological Factors

- Our following presentation of Herbert's model of ASD (Herbert & Weintraub, 2012) will consider in greater depth the interactions among psychological stress, neuroinflammation, oxidative stress, the immune system, and allostatic load.
- Of particular relevance at this point is McEwen's (McEwen & Tucker, 2011) work, which emphasizes that the mediators of stress—including psychological stress, cortisol, sympathetic and parasympathetic responses, inflammatory and anti-inflammatory cytokines, oxidative stress, and immune function—form a network and interact in a nonlinear way possibly contributing to the development of allostatic load.
- Furthermore, McEwen and Tucker (2011) suggest that this network for the stress response provides a pathway through which psychosocial stress may interact with toxins and lead to allostatic load, thereby increasing the health risks conferred by environmental exposures.

Neuroanatomy

- Davidson and McEwen (2012) note that human research suggests that early life stress leads to structural changes in the brain. In particular, areas of the prefrontal cortex show decreased volume while there is an increase in amygdala volume. Such changes could interfere with the development of emotional regulation which is thought to involve interactions between the prefrontal cortex and amygdala (Davidson & McEwen, 2012; Ochsner & Gross, 2005; Wager et al., 2008). Furthermore, Davidson and McEwen (2012) point out that early hypertrophy of the amygdala caused by early life stress may be followed by later atrophy (Davidson and McEwen, 2012; McEwen, 2006) and that this pattern may occur in autism (Davidson and McEwen, 2012; Tottenham & Sheridan, 2010; Nacewicz et al., 2006; Mosconi et al., 2009).

- Teicher et al. (2003) conclude that early life stress is likely to disrupt the functioning of the cerebellar vermis. Furthermore, Schmahmann (2010) considers the vermis to be part of the limbic cerebellum, an area which he suggests may play a central role in ASD. In addition, in an fMRI study of post-institutionalized children who had been raised in foreign orphanages and adopted, Bauer et al. (2009) found that the children had smaller volume superior-posterior cerebellar lobes, which was related to poorer outcomes on tests of planning and memory.
- In addition, the structure and function of the locus coeruleus-noradrenergic system is regulated by diverse stressors and is considered to play a significant role in stress-related psychiatric disorders (Valentino and Van Bockstaele, 2008)

Neuromodulators and Neurotransmitters

- Chronic stress, especially through the action of glucocorticoids, affects the glutamatergic synapse, alters glutamate neurotransmission, and impairs functioning of the prefrontal cortex (Popoli, Yan, McEwen, & Sanacora, 2011).
- Oxytocin and vasopressin neuropeptide systems have been shown to be affected by early neglect and deprivation in children reared in foreign orphanages and later adopted (Wismer Fries, Ziegler, Kurian, Jacoris, & Pollack, 2005).

Neural Networks/Connectivity

- Acute, uncontrollable stress and chronic stress interfere with synaptic functioning and disrupt emotional regulatory networks leading to decreasing modulation of emotions by the prefrontal cortex and increasing amygdala activity (Arnsten, Mazure, & Sinha, 2012).

Sensory Processing

- Both visual processing (Shackman et al., 2011) as well as complex social information processing, especially through interactions between the prefrontal cortex and amygdala (Bishop, 2007), have been shown to be impacted significantly by stress and anxiety.

Unfortunately, discussion of much significant work, including that of Kinsbourne and Helt (2011), Morgan (2006), and Kliman (2011), linking psychological stress and ASD is beyond the scope of this section. Nonetheless, keeping this brief introductory discussion in mind should assist the reader in recognizing the relationships among the following models. Indeed, while emphasizing different factors, all seem to relate to various aspects of the stress response.

HERBERT MODEL: WHOLE BODY DISORDER/GENES-ENVIRONMENTAL STRESS

Martha Herbert (Herbert & Weintraub, 2012; Herbert, 2005b, 2010a) has reconceptualized autism from a biological systems perspective based on her clinical experience with children and adults with autism, on her research demonstrating white matter enlargement in the brains of children with autism (Herbert et al., 2004), and on recent autism research in general. Herbert (Herbert & Weintraub, 2012) sees autism as a dynamic and potentially reversible disorder involving the whole body, from the genetic and cellular levels to brain functioning, communication, and behavior. Genes confer a vulnerability to developing ASD, and the environment can either amplify or diminish this predisposition. Herbert (Herbert & Weintraub, 2012) emphasizes four environmental factors: stress (both emotional and physical), toxins, food and nutrition, and infectious agents, all forming a web influencing—for better or worse—the whole body's functioning.

Herbert (Herbert & Weintraub, 2012) outlines the decline into autistic functioning as follows: some degree of genetic vulnerability plus increased demands on the whole body from the environment (toxins, infectious agents, poor food, and stress) leads to inflammation and oxidative stress which interfere with the functioning of the glia, including the astrocytes. This produces still more oxidative stress which further impairs glial functioning and leads to an excessive level of neuronal excitation. A tipping point then occurs when the allostatic load (the total load of physical and *emotional* stress) is too great. At this juncture astrocytic networks, which are involved in brain information processing as well as brain network coordination and connectivity, begin to malfunction. This further impaired astrocytic functioning then leads to excessive levels of glutamate, sensory overreactivity, and impaired complex information processing in the brain. Autistic behaviors are the final outcome of this pathway which involves many different interlocking vicious circles, including those formed by anxiety (Herbert & Weintraub, 2012).

As noted above, stress from all sources, including emotional stress, plays a central role in the multiple processes leading to the autistic syndrome, for example, emotional stress can activate microglia which "start causing oxidative stress and sending out immune chemicals—cytokines and chemokines—that promote inflammation" (Herbert & Weintraub, 2012, p. 114–115). Emotional stress and physical stress are intimately connected such that increasing one increases the other, while decreases in either emotional or physical stress lead to decreases in the other (Herbert & Weintraub, 2012). For example, through the actions of CRH (corticotropin-releasing hormone) and the sympathetic nervous system, emotional stress can lead to immune suppression and inflammation in the entire body, including the brain (Herbert & Weintraub, 2012). Likewise, oxidative stress and inflammation can contribute to overexcitability and increased emotional stress (Herbert & Weintraub, 2012).

Herbert considers ASD to be a dynamic state rather than a fixed trait. The child with ASD can show rapid and dramatic, but transient, improvement with factors such as fever or treatment with steroids or certain antibiotics (Herbert & Weintraub, 2012). In addition, Herbert cites Beversdorf's (Narayanan et al., 2010) finding that propranolol, which acts on the noradrenergic system and is used to treat symptoms of anxiety, improves brain connectivity within minutes. She even refers to her perspective as a "whole-body, intense-world view of autism" (Herbert & Weintraub, p. 156) and emphasizes that reducing stress can quickly improve brain connectivity and network functioning (Herbert & Weintraub, 2012). She highlights the work of the Markrams (Markram & Markram, 2010) whose intense world model of autism is discussed below. Herbert focuses on their theory that an overly reactive brain makes the world too intense and promotes autistic behavior. Accordingly, autistic avoidance and social withdrawal symptoms are understood as defenses against overly intense stimulation, anxiety, and overload (Herbert & Weintraub, 2012).

Based on her experience with ASD children and their families over a number of years, Herbert is convinced that a significant number of children with autism can improve dramatically; some can recover completely, reach their full potential, and even display exceptional talents (Herbert & Weintraub, 2012). Herbert's interventions revolve around changing the environmental input to reverse this pathological autistic process by decreasing the overall burden of stress and adding support and resources. She emphasizes that more generic, rather than necessarily autism-specific, interventions are likely to have significant benefits (Herbert & Weintraub, 2012). Essential components of her approach include: good diet and nutrition, minimizing exposure to toxins, eliminating infections as well as promoting gut and immune health, and reducing stress—both sensory and social (Herbert & Weintraub, 2012). Finally, Herbert underlines the importance of parents striving to form a positive relationship with their child. She encourages parents to join in their child's special interests and to try to understand and communicate with their children on a deeper level, for example, searching for hidden reasons and messages behind their often enigmatic behavior and helping the child feel recognized and safe (Herbert & Weintraub, 2012).

PORGES: POLYVAGAL THEORY-NEUROCEPTION/ SAFE OR ENDANGERED?

To survive and develop optimally, humans must be able to process sensory information from both the external and internal environments in order to evaluate risk, distinguish between friend and foe, determine whether an environment is safe or dangerous, and communicate and act in an adaptive way with the social group (Porges, 2004/2011; Porges, 2009; van der Kolk, 2011). Thus this process, which Porges calls neuroception, connects the evaluation of risk with social behavior (Porges, 2004/2011). Also essential to survival is the capacity to react to stressors and maintain homeostatic states which promote the development and well-being of the organism (Carter, Harris, & Porges, 2011). Polyvagal theory describes the evolutionary development of the autonomic nervous system, which is central to all of these processes and, thereby, links the neural circuits responsible for evaluating risk and regulating emotions and social interaction with the neural regulation of basic physiological processes underlying the response to stress and supporting health (Porges, 2004/2011; Porges et al., 1994/2011a; Carter et al., 2011). This theory describes the evolution of three primary behavioral strategies or ways of interacting socially, each of which is supported by distinct pathways of the autonomic nervous system. First, the most primitive involves immobilization or behavioral shutdown in the face of severe threat and is dependent on the unmyelinated branch of the vagus nerve. The second involves mobilization or fight-flight behaviors in the face of danger and depends on the sympathetic nervous system. The third, and most recent, in the face of safety, supports social engagement and communication fostered by vocalization, listening, and facial expressions and depends on the myelinated vagus which promotes calm states by inhibiting the sympathetic nervous system (the "vagal brake") (Porges, 2004/2011). Thus, the social myelinated vagus allows social interactions to regulate stress-related physiological states such that the experience of a safe environment leads to social engagement and a calm visceral state (van der Kolk, 2011). However, with an appraisal of danger or threat, the more primitive autonomic nervous system pathways are recruited instead: first, in response to danger, the sympathetic nervous system with fight-flight behaviors and then, in the face of severe threat, immobilization or freezing (van der Kolk, 2011). Furthermore, Porges (1993/2011) notes that interoception, which involves the processing of sensory information coming from the body's interior, including the organs and bodily processes such as digestion and colic or the blood levels of oxygen and carbon dioxide, also contributes to a sense of safety or danger and threat to survival.

Next, as noted above, neuroception is Porges' term to describe the neural circuits involved in the human subconscious system for the detection of safety and danger (Porges, 2004/2011; Carter et al., 2011; Adolphs, 2006). In addition to the autonomic nervous system, this risk surveillance system involves areas of the temporal cortex, including the superior temporal sulcus and the fusiform gyrus, which evaluate facial expressions, voices, and movements of the body and connect to the amygdala (Carter et al., 2011; Adolphs, 2006; Porges, 2009). In addition, the vagal system has connections with the frontal cortex, including upper motor neurons, and, through connections with the parabrachial nucleus and the locus coeruleus, with the hypothalamus, amygdala, and the insula, as well as with prefrontal and orbitofrontal cortices (Porges, 1994/2011b). Also, the neuromodulator oxytocin plays a prominent role in polyvagal theory, neuroception, and social interactions (Carter et al., 2011; Porges, 1998/2011). The release of oxytocin is associated with a sense of safety and, in turn, promotes pleasurable social engagement and the formation of social bonds (Carter et al., 2011).

Now, let's turn to a more specific consideration of polyvagal theory, neuroception, and autism. Once the process of neuroception, which operates outside of conscious awareness, determines whether people or situations are safe, dangerous, or a threat to life, either prosocial or defensive behaviors result as adaptive responses (Porges, 2004/2011). In order to form social bonds and lasting relationships, we must be able to inhibit defensive strategies and become socially engaged under conditions of safety, for example, with the appearance of a loving caregiver. In addition, with the detection of danger, the approach of others leads to defensive reactions, such as withdrawal or aggressive behavior. For this system to operate effectively, humans must be able to switch rapidly and accurately between prosocial and defensive reactions.

Porges (1994/2011b; Porges, 2004/2011) hypothesizes that polyvagal theory and neuroception help to understand and explain autistic spectrum disorder in a number of ways. First, Porges' model assumes an intact, but functionally disrupted, social engagement system (Porges, 1994/2011b; Porges, 2004/2011). In support of polyvagal theory he raises the possibility that faulty neuroception, an inability to assess accurately whether the environment is safe or dangerous or a person is trustworthy or not, may be at the heart of the psychopathology of children with autistic spectrum disorder, as well as those with reactive attachment disorder (Porges, 2004/ 2011). Thus, defensive behaviors may occur in safe environments, and social engagement behaviors may occur in risky environments (Porges, 2004/2011). Next, he suggests that a deficit in the vagal brake leading to an inability to switch between neurobiological states supporting either social or defensive behaviors may be associated with autism (Porges, 1994/2011b).

Third, the social engagement system depends upon autonomic regulation of the muscles of the face and head which subserve gaze direction, eye contact, vocal intonation and rhythm, auditory processing and distinguishing the human voice from sounds in the background, and responsive facial expressions, all of which are commonly disturbed in children with ASD (Porges, 1994/2011b; Porges, 2004/2011). These muscles collectively "function as filters that limit social stimuli (e.g., observing facial features, listening to the human voice)" and as "determinants of engagement with the social environment" (Porges, 1994/2011b, p. 220). With the neuroception of safety comes behavior conducive to social engagement: making eye contact, making contingent facial expressions, vocalizing with appropriate rhythm and inflection, and a greater ability to distinguish the human voice from background sounds (Porges, 2004/2011). The neuroception of danger or threat (whether from an internal or external source) leads to decreased tone in these muscles and to difficulties which are common features of ASD, "difficulties with gaze, extraction of the human voice, facial expression, head gesture, prosody, and state regulation" (Porges, 1994/2011b, p. 221).

Fourth, in addition to the social, emotional, and communication difficulties commonly found in ASD, Porges proposes that neuroception and polyvagal theory also help explain a number of other dysfunctions frequently associated with ASD (Porges, 1994/2011b). The autonomic nervous system and other components of the social engagement system, especially the vagus nerve, are involved in the regulation of the HPA axis, the immune system, and the gastrointestinal system and, thus, could play a significant role in their dysfunction in ASD (Porges, 1994/2011b).

MARKRAM-RINALDI-MARKRAM/PERRY-SZALAVITZ MODEL: INTENSE WORLD-EARLY DEPRIVATION

Szalavitz and Perry (2010) draw together two primary strands in their development of an informal working model of ASD. First, they draw on the Intense World theory formulated by Markram, Rinaldi, and Markram (2007) based on their extensive research involving the valproic acid (VPA) rat model of autism including molecular, cellular, synaptic, microcircuit, and behavioral results. Second, Perry draws on many years of experience involving therapeutic work with maltreated and traumatized children utilizing the principles of neurodevelopment and of the neurobiology of deprivation and other forms of trauma (Perry, 2006). As do Helt et al. (2008) as noted above, Szalavitz and Perry (2010) emphasize that symptoms of early deprivation, including difficulties with empathy and social interactions, sensory problems, extreme tantrums, and repetitive self-soothing behaviors, show a great deal of similarity to ASD. Again, as do Helt et al. (2008), they understand difficulties in ASD to have a neurobiological basis which leads to the developmental (including psychological) experience of deprivation of pivotal early social interactions (Szalavitz & Perry, 2010). The VPA rat model of ASD based on in-utero exposure to VPA has been extensively studied (Markram et al., 2007; Markram et al., 2008; Rinaldi, Perrodin, & Markram, 2008; Markram, 2010). VPA-treated rats, like children with ASD, show impaired social interaction and exploration, increased repetitive behavior, increased anxiety, and decreased habituation to sensory stimuli (Markram, 2010; Markram & Markram, 2010). These rats also show "hyperfear," that is, overgeneralized and enhanced fear memories as well as impaired fear extinction for conditioned fear memories (Markram et al., 2008; Markram et al., 2007). Markram et al. (2007) propose a unifying hypothesis of ASD where the core neurophysiological pathology is hyper-reactivity and hyper-plasticity of microcircuits of the brain with excessive neuronal information processing and storage in local circuits in different brain areas. This causes hyper-functioning of the affected brain regions and, depending upon which area is affected, leads to hyper-attention, hyper-perception, and hyper-memory. This hyper-functioning of certain brain microcircuits, associated with decreased connectivity with other microcircuits, is considered to lead to an experience of the world as painfully intense and fragmented when the neocortex is engaged. This intense world becomes excessively stressful and aversive with the involvement of the amygdala and leads to the experience of social cues as not only overly intense and fragmented, but also frightening. Decreased eye contact, social avoidance and withdrawal, along with repetitive behavior and insistence on routines and sameness are considered to be attempts at coping (Markram et al., 2007; Markram, 2010; Markram & Markram, 2010). However, they also note that the same hyper-functioning neural circuits can lead to exceptional talents (Markram, 2010; Markram & Markram 2010; Markram et al., 2007).

Szalavitz and Perry (2010) concur that sensory overload, heightened fear, and increased stress could lead to some ASD symptoms, including social withdrawal and impaired interactions, as well as repetitive behavior. This leads to a deprivation of key social experiences necessary for development. Without social experiences, which use and exercise the neurons and pathways of the social brain, this brain network atrophies like a muscle. They conclude that, as with neglected children, extreme stress and deprivation of timely appropriate social stimulation may be the cause of social problems seen in ASD. They also postulate that this lack of developmentally appropriate stimulation could be the basis for impaired language development in ASD. Finally, they conclude that, as Perry's work with severely deprived children has demonstrated, what may appear to be fixed, unchangeable deficiencies can, in at least some children, be remarkably open to change with truly intensive treatment. ASD can even perhaps be prevented by early intervention (Szalavitz & Perry, 2010).

MEHLER-PURPURA MODEL: LOCUS COERULEUS-NORADRENERGIC SYSTEM

Mehler and Purpura (2009) postulate that "the dramatic fluctuations in behavioral states occurring during febrile episodes suggest the involvement of a pervasive neural system that can effect relatively rapid changes in the functional activity of widespread neural networks involved in the core features of ASD" (p. 389). Furthermore, Mehler and Purpura (2009) hypothesize that the locus coeruleus-noradrenergic (LC-NA) system, a widespread neuromodulatory system producing and transporting "all of the noradrenaline in the cerebral cortex and hippocampus and most of the NA in other parts of the neuraxis including the cerebellum" (p. 389), represents such a system. The LC-NA system receives diverse input from afferents from "the cerebral cortex, amygdala, basal forebrain and hypothalamus that provide integrated feedback modulation based on evolving environmental contingencies" (p. 389). Overall the LC-NA system is involved in reactions to physiological and environmental stressors (Van Bockstaele et al., 2001) and in responses to salient stimuli. It is also related to behavioral flexibility and to survival in the midst of rapid environmental changes (Bouret & Richmond, 2009). The LC-NA system "seems to be especially related to primitive behavioral reactions that occur when an animal detects a significant change in its environment" (Bouret & Richmond, 2009, p. 910).

Furthermore, the LC-NA system "has been implicated in the etiology of post-traumatic stress disorders" (Mehler & Purpura, 2009, p. 390). They postulate that this system is common to both fever and the modulation of autistic symptoms and that these behavioral changes result from normalization of functional impairments of the LC-NA system. Thus, core autistic symptoms are seen to be the result of developmental dysregulation of a functionally intact LC-NA system which is transiently restored by fever in the following way. LC-NA-hypothalamic pathways are activated by fever and this is thought to lead to activation of the entire LC-NA system and thence to temporary improvement in ASD symptoms (Mehler & Purpura, 2009).

In addition, Mehler and Purpura (2009) postulate that LC-NA dysregulation is the result of epigenetic mechanisms and complex gene-environmental interactions. They cite the above-mentioned study by Kinney et al. (2008a) in which prenatal stress, that is, maternal exposure to hurricanes and tropical storms, resulted in a significant increase in autism prevalence which, furthermore, showed a dose-response effect related to storm severity. High levels of maternal stress could affect the fetal LC-NA system regulation and alter early attachment learning (Mehler & Purpura, 2009; Moriceau & Sullivan, 2005) and possibly interfere with the infant's early sense of safety (Hofer & Sullivan, 2001; Sullivan, 2003).

In conclusion, the symptomatic improvement seen in ASD symptoms during fever could be seen to be related to an increased sense of safety. Therefore, Fischbach's (2010) suggestion that enhanced release of oxytocin and vasopressin from hypothalamic neurons (which send afferents to the locus coeruleus) during febrile episodes could be especially relevant and provide a significant addition to Mehler and Purpura's (2009) LC-NA system model.

DAWSON MODEL: RISK FACTORS-RISK PROCESSES-OUTCOME/ SOCIAL MOTIVATION HYPOTHESIS

The Dawson model proposes that *risk factors* (genetic, phenotypic, and environmental, including toxins and viruses) confer vulnerability to developing ASD by contributing to atypical development of brain and behavior (Dawson, 2008). These risk factors can lead to *risk processes* which heighten underlying vulnerabilities. An altered pattern of child-environment interactions is considered to be a crucial risk process. Such altered interactions with the environment interfere with the child's experiencing essential social and prelinguistic input and result in functional environmental deprivation. This deficiency hinders the development of social and linguistic brain circuits, further amplifying the effects of early risk factors (Dawson, 2008). Thus, in Dawson's model, risk factors interact with risk processes to promote the development of the full syndrome of ASD. Dawson postulates that the full ASD syndrome may not only be treated, but perhaps in certain cases, be prevented by early interventions which focus on these central risk processes, primarily altered child-social environment interactions. Successful early intervention would lead to growth-promoting patterns of interaction between the child and caregivers and, thereby, create an enriched environment having the capacity to lessen the adverse effects of genetic and environmental risk factors (Dawson, 2008).

A central factor in Dawson's model is the social motivation hypothesis. The numerous impairments seen in ASD involving reduced social engagement, such as difficulties with face processing, are considered to be secondary to a fundamental impairment in social motivation which leads to decreased attention to and engagement with people (Dawson, 2008; Dawson et al., 2005). Furthermore, impairments in social motivation may be related to difficulties in the social reward system as outlined below (Dawson, 2008; Dawson et al., 2005). Social reward is understood to play a major role in the development of social brain circuits. Oxytocin and vasopressin are seen to promote prosocial behavior through their activation of the dopamine reward system. This system includes the prefrontal cortex and amygdala and promotes the neural processing of social cues through development of a preference for social stimuli, which involves anticipatory pleasure. This process leads to optimal development of social brain circuits, including the superior temporal sulcus, fusiform gyrus, and language regions and to the development of integrated neural systems subserving such basic social processes as joint attention, social imitation, and intentional communication (Dawson, 2008; Dawson et al., 2005). Finally, effective early interventions which focus primarily on developing adaptive child-environment interactions are considered to operate through increasing social motivation (Dawson, 2008).

Of great significance, Dawson's work played a major role in the development of the Early Start Denver Model, a comprehensive developmental behavioral intervention for toddlers and young children (12–60 months) with ASD (Rogers & Dawson, 2010). A randomized clinical trial indicated that this early behavioral intervention resulted in improvements in social behavior which was associated with normalized patterns of brain activity in young children with ASD (Dawson & McEwen, 2012).

GREENSPAN MODEL: DEVELOPMENTAL, INDIVIDUAL–DIFFERENCE, RELATIONSHIP-BASED DIR/FLOORTIME MODEL

In 1992, Greenspan proposed a model in which ASD does not result from a fixed biological defect in the capacity to form emotional relationships. Rather, differences in areas such as sensory reactivity, sensory processing, and motor tone and motor planning interfere with communication and the formation of interactive relationships and predispose individuals to idiosyncratic and stereotyped behaviors (Greenspan, 1992). The interaction of multiple neurobiological pathways which all contribute to a cumulative risk lies at the heart of Greenspan's understanding of ASD (Greenspan & Shanker, 2004; Greenspan & Wieder, 2006). A number of genetic factors, along with prenatal and postnatal processes, are understood to contribute to the child's cumulative risk of developing ASD. Such factors operate at neurochemical, neurophysiological, and neuroanatomical levels and may involve vulnerabilities to environmental challenges such as toxins and viral infections. In addition, physical or experiential stress may contribute to the manifestations of ASD (Greenspan & Shanker, 2004; Greenspan & Wieder, 2006). These neurobiological factors all lead to what Greenspan (Greenspan & Shanker, 2004; Greenspan & Wieder, 2006) considers to be the "core psychological deficit in autism . . . an inability to connect emotions and intent to motor planning and sequencing and to emerging symbols" (Greenspan & Shanker, 2004, p. 299) as well as to other processing capacities, for example, auditory and visual-spatial—the Affect Diathesis Hypothesis. This core deficit interferes with the child's ability to become affectively connected to and engaged with caregivers in critical purposeful interactions, which further impairs the child's development of fundamental capacities which underlie attuned, empathic communication and warm, pleasurable relationships (Wieder, Greenspan, & Kalmanson, 2008). Greenspan and Wieder (2006) note that children with ASD may become easily overwhelmed by their emotions, and avoid contact with others in their attempts at self-regulation. Furthermore, Greenspan and Shanker (2004) draw a distinct parallel between children with the neurobiologically based syndrome of ASD and the effects of severe emotional deprivation in early life.

Greenspan and others (Greenspan, 1992; Greenspan & Wieder, 1998; Greenspan & Shanker, 2004; Greenspan & Wieder, 2006; Wieder et al., 2008) have developed a comprehensive and multidisciplinary intervention program which is based on a developmental approach to forming interactive relationships with caregivers and which also addresses the child's individual differences in processing and organizing experiences. This intervention program, referred to as the Developmental, Individual-Difference, Relationship-Based DIR/Floortime Model, attempts to reverse the above pathological sequence. Therapists and parents take into account the young child's unique neurobiology and work to create situations of heightened affect and desire in order to motivate the child to "take purposeful action, exchange emotional signals, and interact with others" (Greenspan & Wieder, 2006, p. 397). As a result of such interactions, the child's capacity for motor planning and his ability to interact in a meaningful way improve (Greenspan & Wieder, 2006). By focusing on the development of basic functional emotional capacities the child is helped to resume a healthy developmental trajectory (Wieder et al., 2008). In fact, as a result of such interventions, Greenspan has found short-term changes in engagement and interaction by the end of the first DIR/Floortime consultation (Greenspan & Wieder, 2008). In addition, in a long-term follow-up study involving a chart review of 200 cases of children with ASD who were treated with the DIR/Floortime approach, Greenspan and Wieder (1997) found that 58 percent made "good to outstanding" progress on such criteria as development of a sense of self and relating with warmth and empathy, and were no longer in the autistic range on the Childhood Autism Rating Scale (CARS).

RAMACHANDRAN MODEL: MIRROR NEURON DYSFUNCTION-SALIENCE LANDSCAPE THEORY

Ramachandran has proposed that the mirror neuron system, a large interconnected circuit which includes small groups of cells in many brain regions, evolved in order to form internal models of others' actions and intentions as well as to develop self-representations and self-awareness (Ramachandran, 2011; Ramachandran and Oberman, 2006; Oberman & Ramachandran,

2007). Furthermore, he proposes that the functions of mirror neurons, including empathy, understanding others' feelings, actions and intentions, imitation, and the use of language for social communication are disrupted in ASD because of a potentially reversible dysfunction in the mirror neuron system (Ramachandran, 2011; Ramachandran & Oberman, 2006; Oberman & Ramachandran, 2007).

However, in an earlier attempt to explain other important symptoms of ASD, including repetitive and self-stimulating movements, the insistence on sameness and routine, auditory hypersensitivity, and gaze aversion, Ramachandran (Hirstein et al., 2001; Ramachandran & Oberman, 2006; Ramachandran, 2011) developed "salience landscape theory." He recently noted that there are possible interactions between the mirror neuron system and the neural pathways involved in "salience landscape theory" (Ramachandran, 2011). According to this theory, sensory information is relayed to the amygdala for "emotional surveillance" of the environment and a determination of its potential significance, for example, "is this friend or foe, safe and helpful or dangerous and threatening?" This evaluation passes from the amygdala to other parts of the limbic system, the hypothalamus and the autonomic nervous system, as well as to the frontal lobes, in preparation for an appropriate response. Eventually, a "salience landscape" which details the emotional significance of things in one's world is created by the amygdala (Ramachandran & Oberman, 2006; Ramachandran, 2011). Furthermore, he hypothesizes that because of problems with connectivity between the sensory cortex and the amygdala or between limbic structures and the regulatory frontal lobes, children with ASD have a malfunctioning autonomic nervous system and develop a distorted salience landscape. Therefore, objectively trivial events may lead to extreme autonomic and emotional responses referred to as "autonomic storms" (Ramachandran, 2011). Thus, a child with ASD may prefer sameness and routine and engage in self-stimulating behavior to calm sympathetic autonomic nervous system hyperactivity (Hirstein et al., 2001). In fact, Ramachandran and his group found that children with ASD had a higher overall level of autonomic arousal (measured by GSR) and not only became agitated by trivial events but often ignored stimuli to which normal children had responded in an expected manner (Hirstein, Iversen, & Ramachandran, 2001; Ramachandran & Oberman, 2006). This work led Hirstein to develop a potential treatment for ASD, a portable device to monitor the child's GSR, and, in response to autonomic arousal, activate another device, for example, a "squeeze vest," to provide comforting body stimulation by gently tightening around the child (Ramachandran & Oberman, 2006).

In addition, the psychological aspects of this theory are of potential significance. "Salience landscape theory" concerns the process by which a child determines what is comforting or threatening, what one values and approaches or finds aversive and avoids. Thus, the authors propose that because of autonomic dysfunction, either hyper- or hypo-arousal, children with ASD do not learn that others are of interest and valuable and, in fact, learn to avoid what is vital (Hirstein et al., 2001).

Finally, Ramachandran proposes that "salience landscape theory" may help explain the improvement some ASD children show in response to fever. Because the pathways involved in "salience landscape theory" and autonomic overarousal, that is, the hypothalamus and autonomic nervous system, overlap with those of the temperature-regulatory system, a potential way exists for fever to have a favorable effect on the symptoms of ASD (Ramachandran, 2011).

OCHSNER-ZAKI MODEL: PROCESSING COMPLEX SOCIAL INFORMATION

In a recent series of articles, Ochsner and Zaki (Zaki et al., 2009; Zaki & Ochsner, 2009; Zaki, Hennigan, Weber, & Ochsner, 2010; Zaki & Ochsner, 2011; Zaki & Ochsner, 2012) have increasingly related their social cognition research concerning perceiving and understanding the minds of others to autistic spectrum disorder. In doing so, they have brought together two theories which are each involved both in trying to understand the neural foundations of empathy and in trying to explain central aspects of the autism syndrome, that is, difficulties in understanding what others are feeling, thinking, and intending as well as difficulties in communication and language. Heretofore, these two theories have primarily been kept separate from one another (Zaki & Ochsner, 2011). These theories are (a) the mindblindness theory or delayed development of Theory of Mind (Baron-Cohen, 1995; Baron-Cohen, 2009) and (b) the mirror-neuron hypothesis (Gallese, 2006; Ramachandran, 2011; Oberman & Ramachandran, 2006; Oberman & Ramachandran, 2007). In addition, they have recently begun to explore the associated area of the effects of oxytocin on social cognition as well as prosocial behavior in humans (Bartz et al., 2010b; Bartz et al., 2011).

First, Zaki and Ochsner (2011) describe the Theory of Mind hypothesis as understanding others by attributing mental states to them and utilizing these in social interactions. They refer to this process as mental state attribution and describe a "mental state attribution system" (MSAS). This is considered to be a functional neural network including the medial prefrontal cortex, temporoparietal junction, posterior cingulate cortex, and temporal poles, which is involved in both appraisal of and making decisions about the internal states of others (Zaki & Ochsner, 2011).

They also describe a "shared representations system" (SRS) which refers to the phenomenon of neural resonance—the perceiver's sharing the internal state of an observed other, including motor, sensory, and affective experiences (Zaki & Ochsner, 2011; Zaki et al., 2009). The SRS is considered to be a functional system involving the mirror neuron system and including many different areas of the brain depending upon the internal state of the person being observed, that is, premotor, inferior frontal and inferior parietal cortex; somatosensory cortex; anterior insular and anterior cingulate cortex; and the hippocampus and posterior medial frontal cortex (Zaki & Ochsner, 2011). Zaki and Ochsner (2011) point out that while these two processes and systems both have the same goal (sharing and understanding the internal states of others) the SRS and the MSAS involve almost completely non-overlapping areas of the brain. However, they note that naturalistic, complex social information, unlike the usual laboratory methods, contains both nonverbal (SRS) and contextual (MSAS) information and would be likely to engage both of these systems (Zaki et al., 2010; Zaki & Ochsner, 2011). Indeed, recent research has demonstrated that when responding to complex social information, both of these systems interact, and this interaction contributes to empathic accuracy (Zaki et al., 2009; Zaki & Ochsner, 2009; Zaki et al.2010; Zaki & Ochsner, 2011).

They note several implications for our understanding of ASD and ASD research and treatment. First, considering ASD to involve either dysfunction of the mirror neuron system or deficits in Theory of Mind is too simplistic (Zaki & Ochsner, 2009b). Instead, children with ASD may have difficulty integrating complex, multimodal social information due to abnormal patterns of connection and difficulty with concurrent engagement of multiple neural systems (Zaki & Ochsner, 2011). Therefore, there is a need for research involving more naturalistic social cognitive tasks to study ASD and for the use of measures of performance such as empathic accuracy (Zaki et al., 2009a; Zaki et al., 2010; Zaki & Ochsner, 2011).

Finally, Bartz et al. (2010a) found that in healthy subjects, intranasal oxytocin improves empathic accuracy, but only for individuals who have higher scores as measured by the Autism Spectrum Quotient and are less proficient socially. Furthermore, Bartz et al. (2011) suggest that administered oxytocin can be considered to alter the basic processing of social information, for example, the salience of interpersonal cues, and that the behavioral effects would depend upon features of the situation and/or individual factors.

CONCLUSION

We hope that our brief neurobiological summary has made a worthwhile contribution to understanding how biological and psychological processes are intricately intertwined in ASD. Looking at autism through the lens of the experience of early deprivation, stress, and allostatic load could help to build bridges and promote collaboration between researchers and clinicians. Early deprivation and stress seem to form part of a complex network of biological and psychological factors contributing to the development and maintenance of the ASD syndrome. If the psychological experience of early deprivation, resulting in excessive stress and allostatic load, plays a crucial role in an ongoing pathological process underlying ASD, then one would predict that ameliorating these same factors would lead to improved functioning in children with ASD. This prediction is consistent with the literature review by Helt et al. (2008), who concluded that successful psychosocial intervention using behavioral techniques indeed reverses deprivation and decreases stress and anxiety (Helt et al., 2008).

Psychoanalytic treatment similarly promotes social and emotional engagement, as well as reducing anxiety, and hypothetically could lead to neuroplastic changes and consequent improvement in the ASD syndrome. In fact, analytic dyadic therapy with toddlers which focuses on the parent-child interaction could conceivably bring about positive changes in brain function, as has been shown for the Early Start Denver Model (Dawson et al., 2012). Hopefully, this book can help generate the collaboration and research necessary to test these hypotheses. However, we are optimistic that our clinical material has demonstrated that psychoanalytic understanding and treatment can also effectively address these same areas in ASD children. As we have shown, such analytic work can help the autistic child feel a sense of safety with people and be more lovingly engaged in relationships. Thus, we have attempted to present a plausible basis for linking the psychoanalytic and neurobiological perspectives on autism. Such psychoanalytic work with ASD children might actually facilitate the connection between the "thinking" and the "feeling" parts of the brain (Sherkow, 2007).

Discussion

> Metaphor is now viewed as an emergent property of mind. Metaphor is rooted in the body in two senses: metaphor is used to organize bodily sensation cognitively, especially affects, and secondly, metaphor is rooted in the body as it rests on the border between mind and brain.
>
> —Modell, 1977, p. 105

This book also "rests on the border between mind and brain." It was written by psychoanalysts who have successfully used their psychoanalytic understanding of development to treat children with autism spectrum disorder (ASD). The authors were motivated to share with the therapeutic community the knowledge they have gained both from their study of the research on ASD and particularly from their experiences with their child patients and their families. The essence of what the authors have learned can be summarized by three main ideas. The first is that ASD is a neurodevelopmental disorder that is highly heritable and most likely derives from a heterogeneous group of genetic and epigenetic factors, but is best described as an emergent property of a complex developmental process. The second is that the treatment of ASD should begin as early as possible in the child's life, should include an intensive relationship-based treatment that focuses on making meaning of the child's affective experience of his world (features of psychoanalysis), and should involve the parents. Finally, the third is that with such a treatment, many children with ASD make significant improvements and can even become asymptomatic, representing underlying changes in the brain (Kandel, 1983).

THE NEUROBIOLOGY OF AUTISM SPECTRUM DISORDER

We have provided a highly selective summary of the neurobiological research in the area of ASD. This summary attempts to provide the reader with a grasp of how neurobiological and psychological factors are intermingled in ASD, underscoring our main thesis that ASD is a potentially reversible neurodevelopmental disorder with experiential/psychological consequences. We bring together some of the research on ASD, and the way altered neurobiological functioning impacts the child's emotional development: in particulr its impact on the meanings a young child makes of his or her life experience. In so doing, we lay the groundwork for an integrated treatment approach with psychoanalysis at its core.

Herein we describe ASD as a complex, heterogeneous neurodevelopmental disorder involving multiple genes and biological mechanisms, leading to the disruption of brain circuits mediating language, behavioral flexibility, and social engagement. Much of the research focuses on disordered functioning of the social brain, interfering with pleasurable experience and comforting in the parent-child relationship. In one hypothetical model, neuroinflammation is thought to interfere with neural connectivity and cause social withdrawal and increased stress, which in turn can increase neuroinflammation, in a vicious cycle. In another model, disturbances in the white matter are thought to weaken connections between the prefrontal cortex and other brain regions, impeding integrative functioning and—in conjunction with increased connectivity within the frontal lobe—contributing to hypersensitivity to sensory stimulation.

Our tentative working model indicates the many paths that are correlated with particular biological and environmental factors in ASD—neurobiology including genetic/epigenetic, neuroanatomical, and sensory factors, which are correlated with impaired processing of the social brain, in turn correlated with impaired child/parent interactions/threat, then correlated with psychological conflict and obstruction of social functioning, and finally correlated with ASD symptoms. We emphasize the correlative relationship between these various factors and ASD symptoms, because there are no known direct causal relationships in autism. The neurobiological factors that in some children interfere with the infant's experience of dependable loving and regulating caretaking, as well as distort the trajectory of healthy development are also frequently identified in non-symptomatic siblings. Yet when a child proceeds down a problematic path, it becomes increasingly difficult over time to correct the distortion. The repetition of aversive experience, and the loss of opportunities to learn and master, further burdens the child's relationship to the environment—especially the social environment—impairing the development of a Theory of Mind and associated competencies such as empathy and impulse control. The consequent intensification of the difficulties managing aggression, intimacy, and sexuality can engender extreme conflict in the ASD child, most of all in the parent-child relationship.

More than thirty years ago, Eric Kandel proposed the then revolutionary idea that neuroplastic changes underlie the therapeutic action of psychotherapy (Kandel, 1983). Since then, the capacity of neurons to change in structure and alter their connections to one another as the brain adapts to experience over time has been the subject of considerable neurobiological research, as has the relationship between neuroplasticity and psychotherapy.

We are proposing a model of therapy directed at understanding the subjective experience of the child and using as its focus of intervention the child's important relationships—primarily parent/child, but also relationships with the analyst and collaborating therapists, teachers, and peers. According to this model, what has been a missing element in behavioral therapies—the inner world of the child, its meanings, and the conflicts within it—is brought into the forefront of the therapeutic activity that we believe also can change the brain.

THE CLINICAL CASES

The book centers around the clinical cases, which bring alive the therapeutic work, describing each child's behavior at the onset of the treatment and the process by which the behavior changed in response to the child's increasing capacity to engage with the social world and recognize and make sense of his affective experience. A significant part of this engagement relied on the establishment of a trusting and dependent connection to the analyst and also—crucially—to the parents, allowing the child to find safety and comfort in human relationships. As this capacity grew, the analysts helped the child and the parents to make sense of his own emotions and those of others, discovering the motivation for his and others' behaviors. An essential piece of this work in all the cases involved the tolerance, regulation, and transformation of aggression. The analyst's help in recognizing and making sense of aggressive conflict, which particularly in the case of these children—whose regulatory balance was so easily tipped into often frightening organismic chaos—was a driving factor in relieving their distress and problematic behavior. This work was accomplished through an assortment of symbolic—in words and play—and non-symbolic means. The analyst's acceptance of a central role in the child and family's life, and the respectful and effective use of this role, was foundational in each case.

Age at Onset of Treatment

All the cases presented were in the toddler or preschool age group when they began treatment. Johnny was referred at age 30 months, Dahlia at 42 months,

Corey at 25 months, and Ethan at 28 months. As we have made clear, and as many others have also stressed, the earlier one can intervene with a vulnerable child, the more likely one achieves a positive outcome. In children with ASD, the interplay between the child and his caregiving and physical environment takes place over time. When children with highly sensitive sensory perceptual systems engage with their environments in noxious ways, they create increasingly maladaptive ways of protecting themselves from the ongoing traumatic exposures, and their relationships with their caregivers become more and more distorted and painful. Concurrently, the child is building a sense of himself and of his relationship to the world. In this "inner world" of the child, representational patterns are organized in response to his experience that reflect both his lack of competencies in affect and cognitive processing, and also his defensive operations—such as extreme avoidance—that in turn creates progressive constraints on his continuing growth and development. Thus, although development is essentially unpredictable, intervention that can diminish these constraints as early as possible is advantageous both from the neurodevelopmental and the psychological points of view.

ASD Symptoms in the Cases

All of the children had similar ASD symptoms. Johnny demonstrated the symptoms of twirling, gaze avoidance, and compulsive, stereotyped behaviors. He would bang his head and have temper tantrums. Although he had initially been a cuddly baby, Johnny began to withdraw in his second year of life, when language is developing. His language was delayed, and he had difficulty expressing his needs or emotions. The parents of 3-year-old Dahlia described her as "hard to reach" from the beginning and "lacking emotion and empathy." Her teacher said that Dahlia was unresponsive to adult direction, uninvolved with her peers, sometimes behaving in bizarre and even dangerous ways in the classroom, such as climbing on furniture. Corey had not yet developed babbling or pointing, made no social gestures nor had consistent eye contact, was unresponsive to his name, requests, and directions, and seemed interested in toys only for their mechanical properties but not for pretend play. Corey appeared to be normal in the first year or so of life, though it is possible that signs of ASD were not recognized earlier in infancy. Ethan had a precocious vocabulary but did not use words to communicate and would not answer to his name. He did not show separation reactions and became hyperfocused on repetitive activities such as putting CDs in and out of machines and playing them. All of these "symptoms" reflect derailments in the developmental pathway.

Distinguishing Features of the Cases

In each case there are interesting features that *distinguish* them from one another and that remind us of the heterogeneity of the ASD diagnosis. In the case of Johnny, there is the interesting factor of his being a twin. The intensity of the aggression generated between twins and the challenges presented to the caregiving environment from birth are well known (Ablon et al., 1986). In the case of Dahlia, there is the issue of Chinese culture and language, the implications of her gender, and the assumption that she would be an only child. Yet, perhaps most important, of all the cases Dahlia had the strongest family history of ASD in that three second-order relatives carried an ASD diagnosis. Ethan was remarkable for his precocious vocabulary and had shown no signs for concern until well into his second year of life. Corey seemed closely tied to his mother and exhibited what initially appeared to be signs of physical affection, but which on closer observation seemed to indicate a lack of recognition of his mother as a separate person. These features distinguished our cases one from the other but did not mitigate the ongoing distortions of their developmental trajectories that led them in a similar direction of diminished social, intellectual, and affective competency.

Complex Meaning of the Symptoms: Developmental Deficits and Efforts at Self-Protection

The symptoms of these children are illustrative both of developmental deficits in ASD and of the child's attempt to comfort or protect himself. Johnny's twirling was an attempt to soothe himself and also constituted—just as did his gaze avoidance and compulsive behaviors—efforts to close out a threatening world. When these attempts failed, he would bang his head and have temper tantrums. Dahlia's inability to identify her own feelings and to communicate them to her parents—and even more so, her withdrawal from them—made it hard for them to "know" her. Her lack of responsiveness to adult direction sometimes created dangerous situations, and her awkward social behavior isolated her from her peers.

Corey's disorganized and sometimes destructive use of toys—corresponding to his controlling possessiveness of his mother—demonstrated a lack of capacity for reciprocity and pretend, while at the same time illustrating a maladaptive attempt to control an out-of-control world. Ethan used his precocious vocabulary to exercise control over the other in an effort to contain the disorder of his inner world, and withdrew from relationships with caregivers into self-stimulating activities with CDs. In each case the child's failure to find adaptive ways of self-regulating, of feeling secure and comfortable in the unpredictable world of objects and events, and of people—who are always unpredictable—led him to fall back on behaviors that only further isolated him and prevented him from engaging in opportunities to grow. As we have pointed out, the symptomatic behaviors kept the child stuck on a developmental pathway that was moving progressively in a problematic direction, preventing the child from gaining new competencies and causing him to fall more and more behind his peers.

Therapeutic Intervention: Regulation, Joint Attention, and Moving Toward Reciprocity

The therapeutic interventions that proved so helpful to these children comprised similar features. First, the analyst worked to help the child regulate his affect, motor activity, and arousal state. In addition, the analyst established joint attention between the child and herself, and—in the cases in which the mother was present—the mother. In all cases the analyst narrated to the child what the child was doing and what she observed to be the focus of the child's interest. Also, the analyst characteristically spoke to the child slowly and in simple language—in the case of children who were verbal, choosing words and phrases spoken by the child. The analyst used exaggerated facial expressions to communicate affects clearly and when she was inviting the child to try imaginary play, she used a "marked" (high pitched or gruff voice) to indicate entry into pretend. These principles are illustrated simply in the case of Dahlia—"In my early work with Dahlia, I spoke and moved my body in simple, repetitive actions to establish rhythms that were predictable and provided an easy opportunity for coordination. I was careful to position myself opposite her so that if she did gaze at me directly she could see my face. I used my face and voice to express affect in an amplified manner. I was careful to follow her lead in the play, and I looked for opportunities to support her initiative." (p. 111)

An example from the case of Ethan is richly elaborated. The analyst sang and played toy instruments. This play—repetitive, rhythmic, motoric, and auditory—would be expected to be highly regulatory (Perry & Hambrick, 2008). It created joint attention since it engaged his interest, and it supported his agency in that Ethan initiated the play. Also, because of his engagement in an interactive process and in the rhythmic structure of the play, it worked toward reciprocity. Yet, this example shows that the play with the musical instruments did more than support regulation, joint attention, and the child's initiative. Following a psychoanalytic theory of differentiation, the play created a pattern of vocal and action exchange that included roles for first two and then three participants and also added verbal identifiers (Dr. S and Mommy and Ethan). In this way, the little boy who started with a self-stimulating repetitive action was brought along a regulating wave of musical play toward a simple but rich and increasingly differentiated interpersonal experience.

As described in the cases, we also use the technique of imitation of the child's activities to gain the child's attention and interest, and to enhance the salience of certain behaviors so that analyst and child (and sometimes mother) had an extended opportunity to create meaning of the child's action.[1] In the case of Johnny, the analyst copied him in rolling the toy vehicles up and down on the rug, while also putting this action into words. As she did this, she watched him to assess his response. In those moments, Johnny did not give evidence of noticing her actions, but subsequently, he began to bring his favorite toys to her office. Perhaps the most significant result of this intervention was that the analyst began to "enter the child's world."—"I entered his physical world. I made the assumption that he had a 'mind,' and I guess I was 'pretending' that this was reciprocal play! Ultimately I was letting him know that I could identify with him" (p. 13). Often we find that our words spoken to the child are as helpful to us in our effort to find meaning in what often appears incomprehensible as they are to our child patients—or perhaps more so.

Practitioners of other established and reputable therapeutic methods for ASD children also use some of these techniques to regulate the child, establish joint attention, support the child's initiative, and work toward reciprocal play.[2] However, psychoanalytic treatment diverges from these other methods in significant ways. One particular approach that we as analysts take that is not typically used in other treatments for ASD children is the consistent reliance on symbolic meaning. From the very beginning, often before the child has achieved the capacity for symbolization, we identify symbolic meaning in our little patients' actions and utterances. Perhaps in part because of our extensive experience—both explicit and implicit—in making sense with symbolic meaning, we recognize fragments of incipient or potential symbols, and verbalize them to the child, the mother, and to ourselves.

In a related fashion, due to our persistent attention to the presence of aggressive conflict, we will see representations of aggressive intention in repetitive or apparently random behaviors with toys. For example, in the case of Dahlia, the analyst noted that the child chose the aggressive dinosaurs to play with and referred to a movie in which a dinosaur broke his horn. In her own mind associating a broken horn to destructive aggression, she stated, "That sounds like a scary movie." Dahlia denied that the movie was scary, but pointed out an elephant with a broken tusk and declared that she was finished playing. Rather than immediately attempting to reengage her in play, the analyst focused on the play interruption, interpreting it as defensive, and said, "Lots of kids don't like broken things because they give them broken feelings." This interpretation of the fear of destructive aggression made in the first individual session with the child is characteristic of a psychoanalytic treatment.

In another example of identifying repetitive play as carrying potential aggressive meaning, the analyst responded to Johnny's back-and-forth play with the cars and trains with remarks such as, "Oh no! Thomas is crashing into me!" even if this were not literally the case. Or, "Oh, no! Now I'm hurt!" which elicited grins from Johnny. It is important to note here that it is not our contention that Johnny had in mind a coherent narrative describing the destructive little train's actions, which could then be "discovered" in his play. Instead, we acknowledge that of many "stories" potentially present but not yet formed in Johnny's mind, we are choosing one and initiating its articulation (Harrison, forthcoming). Then, taking the cue from Johnny's response, we will either proceed in a bit by bit fashion along the "track" of the train story, checking in with Johnny at every step, or we will turn back and make another choice. This truly "co-creative" process is reciprocal, and thus the analyst is not only helping Johnny tell a story, but she is helping him learn *how* to tell one in the context of a reciprocal relationship.

An example of how this "co-creative meaning making" proceeded—also in a helpful way involving the mother—appears in the case of Corey, when he rejected the sound effects his mother and Dr. S made in response to his car and doll play by turning away. "Because I approach children like Corey with the premise that 'everything has meaning' as a way to understand his or her unique subjectivity, I assumed that there was meaning there. However, I was stymied to make sense of what Corey was doing, as though our 'joining him' or 'understanding' interrupted his 'play' and drove him away. But even those explanations invoke 'intentionality'. A third possibility was that there was no intentionality to the 'play behavior' but that he was mimicking play sequences that were part of his speech or occupational therapy, . . . Nonetheless, . . . it still suggested a connection that was being made in a mental representational system, but one that neither mother nor I could identify" (p. 43). Again, it can be seen that—perhaps more important than the particular meaning that is proposed—Dr. S and mother are demonstrating to Corey a way of constructing symbolic meaning in play, and though at this time Corey's action is to turn away, he is indeed taking part in the process (Harrison & Tronick, 2007).

The Clinical Integration of Psychoanalytic and Neurodevelopmental Models

In this volume, we explore how analysts working with ASD children use formulations that emerge from both our psychoanalytic and neurodevelopmental understanding. This point is well illustrated in all four cases.

Johnny

To illustrate the rich use of play and narrative within the relationship to analyst and mother and guided by an integrated theory, consider the example of Johnny and the twin towers. Mother was annoyed at Johnny's "autistic behavior" of repeatedly reciting "chitty chitty bang bang." We can imagine that mother's annoyance was complex and related to her inability to make sense of Johnny's behavior and his lack of responsiveness to her, while always in the background were her frightening fantasies of his future that this "weird" behavior provoked.

Assuming that the behavior did in fact have meaning and was not necessarily weird, the analyst speculated that Johnny's "agitated actions and sing-song voice . . . appeared to be mirroring his mother's anxiety about his autistic behavior." This conjecture finds validation in developmental studies about the communication of affect in the caregiving relationship (Reddy, 2008; Stern, 1985; Trevarthen, 2005).

The psychoanalyst, formulating Johnny's behavior in his repetitive, "chitty chitty bang bang" behavior, states, "At this point he and I both knew that this stereotypic behavior signaled his distress with his mother, his knowledge of her disappointment in him and in *me* because he was still symptomatic, her despair that he was irreparably damaged, and his way of blocking her out and driving her crazy at the same time—his punishment of her for all past and current 'crimes'—all of which I had verbalized at one time or another over the previous few months" (p. 18).

Using the technique of imitation—a technique devised by Johnny's analyst but also described in therapeutic models based on developmental science—she picked up a toy train and began chanting, "chitty chitty bang bang," "mirroring" Johnny's tone of voice. This interrupted Johnny's avoidant behavior and engaged his attention. In this moment of *shared attention*, a central concept in early development, Johnny communicated to the analyst his interest in blocks by standing on the blocks box. She followed his lead and opened it, then began to build a tower for him to knock down. When he appeared hesitant to knock down her tower with the block she offered to him, she knocked it down herself, interpreting his fear of the terrorist attack, "The tower crashed! It was so scary!" Johnny then pulled out a book about a dog hiding from his mother and the analyst interpreted, "You are worried that Mommy will be angry at you for crashing the towers." He then looked directly into her eyes and responded, "Yes." Thus, the analyst drew on her familiarity with the early developmental concepts of nonverbal affective communication, imitation, and joint attention, to create the play context in which she could make psychoanalytic interpretations of his conflicts about aggression and their role in the mother-child relationship.

Ethan

In the case of Ethan, the analyst understood his compulsive attachment to CDs and his mother's credit cards as transitional objects and appreciated his need for help with the developmental task of separation. She pretended to write notes to missing family members such as his daddy or his grandparents to help him build an awareness of important people in his life who were not present in the moment so that he could represent them in his cognitive and psychological world, building a "Theory of Mind" (Baron-Cohen et al., 1995). She used the same technique to prepare Ethan for separations from family members and from her by writing notes about real impending separations and transitions.

The analyst recognized the significance of Ethan's new ability to say "no" to his mother in the context of playing musical instruments, and she elaborated this negativity by creating songs about who could play and who could not, serving to support both his emerging capacity to say "no" and the accompanying capacity for differentiation. This "no" could also be seen as a precursor to his angry insistence on keeping his poopy diaper, and to his checking that his penis was still there when his diaper was changed. In this way, the analyst could use words and play to help Ethan create competencies that he could then use to make sense of other developmental challenges such as toilet training, gender difference, and the fear of the loss of bodily integrity. This psychoanalytic work is not necessarily different from the treatment of children who do not have ASD, but the special challenges presented by the lack of competencies in self-regulation, communication, and social engagement, make it harder and more interesting.

Corey

In the case of Corey, the analyst describes the disturbed relationship Corey had to his mother. Corey would physically throw himself on her but would not communicate with her in language. Corey's mother would not set limits on his behavior and in fact allowed him to behave in ways that put him in potential danger. The analyst formulated that Corey's original neurodevelopmental vulnerability, and perhaps the consequence of his enhanced dependency on her, contributed to his mother's failure to scaffold his separation-individuation. In addition, his mother was influenced by her own character, which interfered with her capacity to recognize her son as a person in his own right and caused her to direct him to "Show Dr. S" this and that, rather than to support his own agenda.

It is difficult to imagine how anything other than a dyadic treatment could affect the necessary changes in this relationship. For example, when the analyst said, "Corey, your mother will let you eat the raisins as long as you eat them without gobbling, and instead, eat them 'one by one'," she was speaking simultaneously to both partners in the dyad. She was communicating the need for order in the context of chaos and at the same time she was offering a *means of restoring order* in her use of the phrase, "one by one," suggesting slowing down and taking one thing at a time.

This intervention might be seen as primarily developmental, since it was regulating and also supported the caregiving function of the relationship. Yet, as we have seen, it was also psychoanalytic, in that it communicated a link between intention (mother's) and behavior (Corey's) and was moving—in the analyst's mind—toward the goal of differentiation. This formulation about defective separation-individuation was further validated by the analyst's visit to the school, where she observed Corey treating other children as if they were inanimate objects. Referring to Baron-Cohen, the analyst remarks that "this was consistent with Baron-Cohen's observation that ASD children have active sensory apparatus but cannot create the triangle of shared experience, Baron-Cohen's "triangulation of joint attention" (p. 59).

A fascinating adjunct to the separation-individuation formulation is presented in Corey and his mother's behaviors when they returned from a week-long vacation to Florida. Both mother and child were so dysregulated on their return to the analyst that it is hard not to interpret their behaviors as "lacking a strategy for reunion," as is the case in disorganized attachment (Hesse & Main, 2000). It should be stressed, however, that the reference to Attachment Theory does not challenge the psychoanalytic formulations used by the analyst in this case—that "Corey was angry at me for having let him go on vacation." Instead, it enriches our understanding by including in the formulation information about the lack of developmental competency in the attachment domain (Fonagy et al., 2002). As the analyst and Corey and his mother continued, the analyst—guided by her psychoanalytic theory of separation-individuation—repeatedly used the name, "Mommy," to enhance his mother's identity as a separate person. Corey then chose to play with blocks, building towers and knocking them down. Here again, one can imagine the simultaneous making of meanings in different domains—the symbolic domain of representing rupture and repair, while in the domain of attachment, creating a *strategy for reunion*—playing in a way that organizes one's aggressive and affective experience.

Dahlia

In the case of Dahlia, the analyst attempted to help her "grow" her play so that it could become less routinized and more open to creative elaboration. In her play, the story basically involved the good guys—who were distinguishable from the bad guys only by the animal Dahlia chose to represent them, and she could give no reason for choosing these particular animals—attacking the bad guys with growls and yells. It seemed as if Dahlia could barely hold herself together in excited anticipation of the attack, before bursting upon the bad guys (Dahlia always insisted that the analyst play the bad guys) in a storm of unmodulated aggression. The aggressive outburst remained undifferentiated, and afterward, Dahlia could not move on to another play scenario, but seemed stuck in repeating the identical attack. There was no explanation of what the bad guys did to make them deserve such an attack and no explanation of how the punishment was chosen or even planned out. The analyst wanted to open up the subject, because she knew that Dahlia sometimes had temper tantrums and displeased her parents and teachers in ways that might make her feel like a "bad guy." She was concerned about the punitiveness of the punishments meted out to the bad guys that, she presumed, Dahlia felt that she herself sometimes deserved.

Though the analyst was thinking in psychoanalytic terms about Dahlia's conflicts about aggression and her punitive superego, she was also aware that Dahlia's cognitive rigidity and fragile affective and physiological arousal would make it hard to address the issue. Each day Dahlia proceeded as usual to set up the scenario on the analyst's library ladder steps, with the "bad guys" occupying the two top steps and the "good guys" entering from the surrounding area and attacking them. When she set up the animals, Dahlia would never look at the analyst, relating to the analyst as if she were a prop in her play. Sometimes the analyst asked her, "What did the bad guys do to make them bad?" She would respond, "I don't know. Let's play." The analyst repeated her question at different times in the play as she was preparing the scene for the attack. Sometimes she would make one of the bad guys start to hatch what she imagined to be a bad guy plan, but Dahlia would never seem to notice and would move in on the bad guys with her good guy attackers, oblivious to anything but the excitement of the ambush.

One day, the analyst stopped in the middle of the play and told Dahlia that she was not going to continue until Dahlia helped her to understand what the bad guys had done to deserve punishment. Dahlia looked at her in surprise and thought about it. She clearly wanted the analyst to play with her, because she needed her to enact this favorite play scenario. Then she pronounced that the bad guys had eaten the good guys' food. After that, Dahlia seemed to enjoy the play even more. While still displaying the intensity of aggression during the attack, Dahlia joined the analyst in playfully elaborating the bad guys' hatching plans to steal the good guys' food. She would say, "Now make them say, 'Oh, those cherries look delicious! Let's take them!'" and the analyst would do as she directed. Unwittingly, the analyst was allowing Dahlia to feel "joined" in expressing her bad behavior, a step toward joint attention. In addition, the process of "joining" allowed Dahlia to elaborate on her heretofore unspoken fantasy of stealing food, and truly "let in" her analyst's empathetic connection. This play elaboration helped Dahlia move in the direction of greater developmental mastery. With her enhanced enjoyment in her play, Dahlia "caught on" to the idea of making the play more fun and interesting by adding complexity and was able—with the analyst's support—to achieve better affective and physiological regulation in the course of her evolving play.

Working with Parents

The authors emphasize that working with the parents is paramount in the successful treatment of these children, since the parents' capacity to empathize with and imaginatively "reach" their children creates the basis for positive experiences in the relationship necessary for learning, and allows the world of human interactions to open up to the children. There is a variety of ways to work with parents. We have found that a particularly effective way of working with parents of very young children is in a dyadic treatment in which the child and parent are seen together by the analyst. In a dyadic treatment, the analyst is aware that all her interventions are received by both parent and child. Although the child's internal life is the focus of the analyst's attention, in some sense it might be said that the parent-child relationship is the patient (Lieberman, Padron, Van Horn, & Harris, 2005).

Johnny's mother was terrified of his diagnosis of ASD and reacted with extreme anxiety and distress when Johnny would exhibit self-stimulating behaviors such as twirling. As the analyst was able to make sense of Johnny's behaviors and communicate her understanding to both Johnny and his mother, Johnny's mother's anxiety about her son diminished, and she became an important ally in the treatment. Corey's mother began with a particularly complicated relationship with the analyst, in which her competition with the analyst for control over her child's life led her to challenge the analyst and devalue her. Nevertheless, as the analysis proceeded, she too became an ally in the crucial process of helping her child become his own person. Ethan's mother quickly came to play an important role in her son's treatment. Finding great comfort and support in her relationship with the analyst, her depression and anxiety diminished, and she was able to contribute insights of her own to the evolving understanding of Ethan's inner world. Dahlia's mother had a particular talent for empathizing with her daughter and for creating opportunities for Dahlia to learn new developmental skills. She was also a tireless advocate for her in the school system, the importance of which we cannot underestimate.

Another effective method for helping parents of ASD children is parent groups. Groups—usually held weekly or even less frequently—do not offer the same intensity of contact with the analyst. However, when they include videotape feedback, as in the case of Dahlia's mother, the opportunity for gaining empathic understanding of the child is profound. The parent's empathic capacity is developed through the observation and analysis of tapes of the parents and their child in interaction. Sharing this activity with other parents is a powerful experience, and parents quickly become adept at videotape analysis. Also, the positive effect of the tolerance and compassion communicated by the other parents can have a remarkable therapeutic effect. Groups are harder for the analyst to run, because analysts are rarely trained in group therapy and less often trained in the use of videotape; also the organization and administration of groups is challenging. Nonetheless, the remarkable benefit of this therapeutic intervention on the parent-child relationship and on the parents' mental health make it an important consideration in treatment planning (Smolen, forthcoming).

Although we have spoken about parent work as occupying a role of central importance, almost all our descriptions of parent work involve the mothers. This is true for the usual reasons—the mother is generally the primary caregiver, the mother is often though not always more available for therapy sessions. And mothers are often the more vocal and insistent parent in the demand for help for their child. This we see as a problem in the treatment of ASD children. It is also is usually indicative of a problematic dynamic in the family, in which the parents become polarized in their feelings and attitudes toward the child who is the source of such pain and conflict in the family. As in the case of Corey, the father often gets pushed to the side, as the mother claims a dominant role in the caregiving; this is an important task for future work.

It is important to acknowledge the pain and fear experienced by both parents of children with ASD. One of the authors describes it in terms of someone longing to dance, but when her dancing partner appears, discovers that he either steps on her feet or drifts away, leaving her hurt and alone. From the earliest days of "refrigerator mothers" to some contemporary psychologies that place responsibility for the child's development on the mother and her "attuned" responses, mothers and fathers of children with ASD have been misunderstood and sometimes mistreated. The authors have stressed the biological origins of ASD and focused their treatments on preparing their child patients to be "dancing partners" who can respond to their parents' caregiving, while at the same time helping the parents appreciate the "why" of their child's problematic behaviors so that they can become increasingly effective in their parenting. When this happens, as another author says, "a spiral upwards" can be created that can move the child toward a healthier developmental trajectory.

WHY PSYCHOANALYSIS?

Since all of these children had multiple simultaneous therapeutic interventions, what is the basis for the authors' emphasis on the psychoanalytic treatment as the primary driver of developmental and therapeutic change? What does psychoanalysis have to offer children with ASD and related developmental disorders?

First, the training and experience of a psychoanalyst is unique in that it involves developing an intimate, dependent relationship with a person in need, with the focus of attention on that individual's inner world and also in the interaction between the two analytic partners. This attention to what is going on in the relationship, in the moment, contributed to by both partners, and understood at a deep level—both symbolically and in the implicit and nonverbal—allows for a different kind of co-creative meaning making. We would consider the capacity to do this to be the unique competence of the psychoanalyst.

Second, psychoanalytic training and experience includes a high degree of "pattern recognition," for example, an ability to recognize symbolic representations of strong emotions within relationships, and combinations and sequences of emotion and psychological efforts at self-protection or defense. Illustrations of these patterns might include a child's remark about a tornado followed by an association to the child's younger brother. Another example might be recognizing that a child attempts to protect him- or herself from threatening aggression coming from within by turning away from the perceived source of the threat, or by retaliating against an imaginary external threat. The capacity for pattern recognition is particularly important in working with ASD children.

Refined pattern recognition also allows the psychoanalytic clinician to take a less linear approach to the treatment of ASD children, in that partial or relatively incoherent symbolic representations are easier to spot and to use in understanding the child's experience and in formulating appropriate communication to the child. This often can be helpful even if the child is not considered to be at a level capable of apprehending such a communication according to other models.

Third, psychoanalytic training and experience requires learning a great deal about oneself. This self-knowledge might include the clinician's personal organizing fantasies, for example, to rescue a suffering child, or the stressors that challenge a clinician's sense of him- or herself, such as making a mistake or causing pain in another person. It also allows the analyst to distinguish between those times when his affective relationship with his patient is neutral compared to those times when his own emotional challenges might play a role.

Psychoanalytic training also allows for a deeper and more comprehensive understanding of parents—how adults cope with stress, how they transmit early relational patterns from one generation to the other, how they grow. Psychoanalysts learn how to tolerate anguished attacks without taking them personally, how to help a suffering person move from the perception of being a victim to that of taking an active role in recovery, and how to move into a collaborative role with another in the context of threat.

Psychoanalysis "off the couch" is valuable not only to the psychoanalytically trained clinician, but to the team that treats these children. We believe that a team that includes specialists in psychoanalysis or psychodynamic psychotherapy, occupational therapy, speech, and education should treat all children with autistic spectrum disorders. Pediatricians or pediatric specialties are also sometimes needed. It is very challenging to organize a team into a collaborative partnership in which roles are clear and compatible and in which there is adequate communication, but it is possible. It is also challenging—though we also believe possible—to make such a comprehensive team approach affordable rather than being an unbearable burden on the parents.

We hope we have succeeded in offering a guidebook to understanding and treating children with ASD or uneven development, especially those who are newly diagnosed, from the dual perspectives of psyche and neurofunction. In sharing with our readers our dyadic work with toddlers and their mothers, and our work with youngsters in a special school setting, we also hope that we have conveyed the insights we have gained about technical considerations, and about mechanisms of change, from our psychoanalytically informed treatments. We believe that the integrative function of a psychoanalytically based therapy can bring a profound understanding of a child's unique internal experience, and of his relationship to his primary caregiver, to any treatment protocol.

NOTES

1. "I began treatment by imitating Susan's movements and speech as closely as possible, rolling on the floor, drawing, or bouncing a ball when she did; essentially, I tried to enter her world. With excruciating slowness she began to take notice of me and to express anger when she felt I was 'doing it wrong.' Perhaps the most dramatic achievement over those two years was her becoming aware of the difference between 'you' and 'me.' Susan went on to many years of treatment with other therapists, including a long stay in a residential treatment center. She is now a young adult and functioning quite well with a job, an apartment of her own. and a boyfriend—able to communicate not only in English but also in German." (p. 61). Interestingly, Chused does not describe this child as ASD; yet, the child's outcome suggests serious developmental problems (Chused, 1988).

2. ESDM, or Early Start Denver Model, based on the Lovaas method of behavioral treatment, also begins by establishing adequate regulation and joint attention. This method focuses on teaching skills, particularly language, and has demonstrated significant improvement in very young ASD children in empirical studies (Rogers, S., "Integrating relational and behavioral approaches to intervention for the youngest children with ASD," Presentation to the U Mass Boston Infant Parent Mental Health Postgraduate Certificate Program, Jan. 26, 2013). DIR, or Relationship-Based Early Intervention Approach to Autistic Spectrum Disorders, also begins with these goals, also emphasizing the child's initiative; it is less focused on training specific skills and more aimed at developing reciprocity and symbolic play (Greenspan & Wieder, 2011).

References

PREFACE

Amaral, D. G., Rubenstein, J. L., & Rogers, S. J. (2008). Neuroscience of autism. In A. Tasman, J. Kay, J. Lieberman, et al. (eds.), *Psychiatry* (pp. 379–392). Chichester, England: Wiley-Blackwell.

Anderson, M., Hooker, B., & Herbert, M. R. (2008). Bridging from cells to cognition in autism pathophysiology: Biological pathways to defective brain function and plasticity. *American Journal of Biochemistry and Biotechnology*, *4*(2), 167–176.

Dawson, G. (2008). Early behavioral intervention, brain plasticity, and the prevention of autism spectrum disorder. *Development and Psychopathology*, *20*(03), 775–803.

Helt, M., Kelley, E., Kinsbourne, M., Pandey, J., Boorstein, H., Herbert, M., & Fein, D. (2008). Can children with autism recover? If so, how? *Neuropsychology Review*, *18*(4), 339–366.

Herbert, M.R. (2005a). Autism biology and the environment. *San Francisco Medicine Journal of the San Francisco Medical Society*, *78*(8), 13–16.

Herbert, M. R. (2005b). Large brains in autism: The challenge of pervasive abnormality. *The Neuroscientist*, *11*(5), 417–440.

Herbert, M. R. (2010). Contributions of the environment and environmentally vulnerable physiology to Autism Spectrum Disorders. *Current Opinion in Neurology*, *23*(2), 103–110.

Herbert, M., & Anderson, M. (2008). An expanding spectrum of autism models: From fixed developmental defects to reversible functional impairments. In A. W. Zimmerman (ed.), *Autism: Current theories and evidence* (pp. 429–463). Totowa, NJ: Humana Press.

Herbert, M. R., & Weintraub, K. (2012). *The autism revolution: Whole-body strategies for making life all it can be*. New York: Ballantine Books.

INTRODUCTION

Baron-Cohen, S. (1995). *Mindblindness: An Essay on Autism and Theory of Mind*. Cambridge, MA: MIT Press.

Baron-Cohen, S., Leslie, A, M and Frith, U. (1985). Does the autistic child have a "theory of mind"? *Cognition, 21*, 37–46.

Barry, V. C. (2000). Reflections on interactive and self-organizing aspects of learning in psychoanalysis. *Annual of Psychoanalysis*, *28*, 7–20.

Carter, A. S., Mayes, L. C., & Pajer, K. A. (1990). The role of dyadic affect in play and infant sex in predicting infant response to the still-face situation. *Child Development, 61*, 764–773. DOI: 10.2307/1130961.

Dawson, G. (2008), Early behavioral intervention, brain plasticity, and the prevention of autism spectrum disorder. *Dev. Psychopathology, 20*, 775–803.

Freud, A. (1962), Assessment of childhood disturbances. *The Psychoanalytic Study of the Child, 17*, 149–158. New York: International Universities Press.

Fonagy, P., Gergely, G., Jurist, E., Target, M. (2002). *Regulation, mentalization, and the development of self.* New York: Other Books.

Fonagy, P., & Target, M. (1998). Mentalization and the changing aims of child psychoanalysis. *Psychoanal. Dial, 8,* 87–114. DOI: 10.1080/10481889809539235.

Harrison, A. M., & Tronick, E. Z. (2007). Contributions to understanding therapeutic change: Now we have a playground. *J. Amer. Psychoanal. Assn., 55*, 853–874.

Helt, M., Kelley, E., Kinsbourne, M., Pandey, J., Boorstein, H., Herbert, M. & Fein, D. (2008). Can children with autism recover? *Neuropsych. Rev., 18*, 339–366.

Herbert, M. R., & Weintraub, K. (2012). *The autism revolution: Whole body strategies for making life all it can be. Harvard Health Publications.* New York: Random House with Harvard Health Publications.

Jacobson, E. (1954). The self and the object world. *Psychoanalytic Study of the Child, 9*, 75–127.

Kliman, G., & contributing editor Burian, E. (2011). *Reflective network therapy in the pre-school classroom*. Lanham, MD: University Press of America.

Klin, A., & Jones, W. (2011). Embodied pscyhoanalysis? Or, on the confluence of psychodynamic theory and developmental science. In *Developmental science and psychoanalysis.* London, Karnac.

Qian, N., & Lipkin, R. M. (2011). A learning-style theory for understanding autistic behaviors. *Frontiers in Human Neuroscience, 5,* 1–17. DOI: 10.3389/fnhum.2011.0007710.3389/fnhum.2011.00077.

Sherkow, S. (2011). The dyadic psychoanalytic treatment of a toddler with autism spectrum disorder. *Psychoanalytic Inquiry*, 31, 252–275.

Sherkow, S. (2005, 2006, 2013). The dyadic psychoanalytic treatment of a toddler with autism spectrum disorder. Presented to the American Psychoanalytic Association, New York, winter meetings.

Sherkow, S. (2013). Lecture at Aaron School, New York.

Singletary, W. (2009). Introduction: Psychoanalytic approaches to autism spectrum disorder: Extending the dialogue between psychoanalysis and neurobiology. Presented to the American Psychoanalytic Association, New York, winter meetings.

Stern, D. N. (2000). *The interpersonal world of the infant: A view from psychoanalysis and developmental psychology*. New York: Basic Books.

Tustin, F. (1988), Psychotherapy with children who cannot play. Internet. *Rev. Psycho-Anal., 15*, 93–106.

Winnicott, D. W. (1956). Primary maternal preoccupation. In *Collected papers: Through pediatrics to psychoanalysis*. London: Tavistock, pp. 300–305.

Winnicott, D. W. (1958). The capacity to be alone. *Int. J. of Psychoanal.* 39, 416–420.

Winnicott, D. W. (1962). Ego integration in child development. *The maturational processes and the facilitating environment* (1965) london: Hogarth, 56–63.

CHAPTERS 1–5

Baron-Cohen, S. (1995). *Mindlbindness: An essay on autism and theory of mind.* Cambridge, MA: MIT Press.

Bergman (2004). Personal communication.

Evered, L. (2011). Neurobiology of aspergers and autism. Presented to Home Alone Association, San Francisco.

Fischbach, G. (2010). Personal communication.

Fonagy, P., & Target, M. (1998). Mentalization and the changing aims of child psychoanalysis. *Psychoanal. Dial., 8*, 87–114. DOI: 10.1080/10481889809539235.
Helt, M. E., Kelley, M., Kinsbourne, J., Pandey, H., Boorstein, M., Herbert, & D. Fein. (2008). Can children with autism recover? *Neuropsych. Rev., 18*, 339–366.
Kliman, G., & contributing editor Burian, E. (2011). *Reflective network therapy in the preschool classroom*. Lanham, MD: University Press of America.
Klin, A., & Jones, W. (2011). Embodied psychoanalysis? Or, on the confluence of psychodynamic theory and developmental science. In *Developmental science and psychoanalysis*. London: Karnac.
Qian, N., & Lipkin, R. M. (2011). A learning-style theory for understanding autistic behaviors. *Frontiers in Human Neuroscience, 5*, 1–17. DOI: 10.3389/fnhum.2011.0007710.3389/fnhum.2011.00077.
Rogoff, B. (2008). Observing sociocultural activity on three planes: Participatory appropriation, guided participation, and apprenticeship. *Pedagogy and Practice: Culture and Identities*, 58–74.
Tustin, F. (1988), Psychotherapy with children who cannot play. *Int. Rev. Psychoanal., 15*, 93–106.

CHAPTERS 6–7

Fonagy, P., Gergely, G., Jurist, E., & Target, M. (2002). *Affect regulation, mentalization and the development of the self.* New York: Other Press.
Greenspan S., & Wieder, S. (2011). Relationship-based early intervention approach to autistic spectrum disorders: The DIR model. In D. G. Amaral, G. Dawson, & D. H. Geschwind (eds.), *Autism Spectrum Disorders* (pp. 1068–1080). New York: Oxford University Press.
Harrison A. M. (2005). Herd the animals into the barn: A parent consultation model of child evaluation. *Psychoanal. Stud. Child, 60*, 128–157.
Harrison A. M., & Tronick, E. Z. (2011). "The noise monitor": A developmental perspective of verbal and nonverbal meaning-making in psychoanalysis. *J. Amer. Psychoanal. Assoc., 59(5)*, 961–983.
Kliman, G., & contributing editor Burian, E. (2011). *Reflective network therapy in the preschool classroom*. Lanham, MD: University Press of America.

CHAPTERS 8–9

Abrahams, B. S., & Geschwind, D. H. (2010). Connecting genes to brain in the autism spectrum disorders. *Archives of Neurology, 67*(4), 395–399.
Adolphs, R. (2006). How do we know the minds of others? Domain-specificity, simulation, and enactive social cognition. *Brain Research, 1079*(1), 25–35.
Amaral, D. G., Rubenstein, J. L., & Rogers, S. J. (2008). Neuroscience of autism. In A. Tasman, J. Kay, J. Lieberman, et al. (eds.), *Psychiatry* (pp. 379–392). Chichester, England: Wiley- Blackwell.
Amaral, D., Schumann, C., & Nordahl, C. (2008). Neuroanatomy of autism. *Trends in Neurosciences, 31*(3), 137–145.
Andari, E., Duhamel, J., Zalla, T., Herbrecht, E., Leboyer, M., & Sirigu, A. (2010). Promoting social behavior with oxytocin in high-functioning Autism Spectrum Disorders. *Proceedings of the National Academy of Sciences, 107*(9), 4389–4394.
Anderson, M., Hooker, B., & Herbert, M. R. (2008). Bridging from cells to cognition in autism pathophysiology: Biological pathways to defective brain function and plasticity. *American Journal of Biochemistry and Biotechnology, 4*(2), 167–176.
Arnsten, A., Mazure, C., & Sinha, R. (2012). This is your brain in meltdown. *Scientific American, 306*(4), 48–53.

Bachevalier, J., & Loveland, K. (2006). The orbitofrontal–amygdala circuit and self-regulation of social–emotional behavior in autism. *Neuroscience & Biobehavioral Reviews, 30*(1), 97–117.

Baron-Cohen, S. (1995). *Mindblindness*. Cambridge, MA: MIT Press.

Baron-Cohen, S. (2009). The empathising-systemising theory of autism: Implications for education. *Tizard Learning Disability Review, 14*(3), 4.

Baron-Cohen, S., Ring, H., & Bullmore, E., et al. (2000). The amygdala theory of autism. *Neuroscience and Biobehavioral Reviews, 24*, 355–364.

Bartz, J. A., Zaki, J., Bolger, N., Hollander, E., Ludwig, N. N., Kolevzon, A., & Ochsner, K. N. (2010a). Oxytocin selectively improves empathic accuracy. *Psychological Science, 21*(10), 1426–1428.

Bartz, J., Zaki, J., Ochsner, K., Bolger, N., Kolevzon, A., Ludwig, N., & Lydon, J. (2010b). Effects of oxytocin on recollections of maternal care and closeness. *Proceedings of the National Academy of Sciences, 107*(50), 21371–201375.

Bartz, J., Zaki, J., Bolger, N., & Ochsner, K. (2011). Social effects of oxytocin in humans: context and person matter. *Trends in Cognitive Sciences, 15*(7), 301–309.

Bauer, P., Hanson, J., Pierson, R., Davidson, R., and Pollack, S. (2009). Cerebellar volume and cognitive functioning in children who experience early deprivation. *Biol. Psychiatry, 66*, 1100–1106.

Begley, S. (2007). *Train your mind, change your brain: How a new science reveals our extraordinary potential to transform ourselves*. New York: Ballantine Books.

Belmonte, M. K., Gomot, M., & Baron-Cohen, S. (2010). Visual attention in autism families: "unaffected" sibs share atypical frontal activation. *Journal of Child Psychology and Psychiatry, 51*(3), 259–276.

Bishop, S. (2007). Neurocognitive mechanisms of anxiety: an integrative account. *Trends in Cognitive Science, 11*(7), 30–316.

Bodfish, J. W. (2011). Repetitive behaviors in individuals with autism spectrum disorders. In D. Amaral, G. Dawson, & D. H. Geschwind, *Autism spectrum disorders* (pp. 200–212). New York: Oxford University Press.

Bouret, S., & Richmond, B. (2009). Relation of locus coeruleus neurons in monkeys to Pavlovian and operant behaviors. *Journal of Neurophysiology, 101*(2): 898–911.

Bryson, S. (2005). The autistic mind. In M. L. Bauman & T. L. Kemper (eds.), *The neurobiology of autism* (pp. 34–44). Baltimore: Johns Hopkins University Press.

Carter, C., Harris, J., & Porges, S. (2011). Neural and evolutionary perspectives on empathy. In J. Decety and W. Ickes (eds.). *The social neuroscience of empathy* (pp.169–182). Cambridge: MIT Press.

Courchesne, E., Webb, S. J., & Schurmann, C. M. (2011). From toddlers to adults: The changing landscape of the brain in autism. In D. Amaral, G. Dawson, & D. H. Geschwind (eds.), *Autism spectrum disorders* (pp. 611–631). New York: Oxford University Press.

Cozolino, L. J. (2002). *The neuroscience of psychotherapy: Building and rebuilding the human brain*. New York: W. W. Norton.

Cozolino, L. J. (2006). *The neuroscience of human relationships: Attachment and the developing social brain*. New York: Norton.

Cozolino, L. J. (2010). *The neuroscience of psychotherapy: Healing the social brain*. New York: W. W. Norton.

Cramer, S., Sur, M., Dobkin, B. H., O'Brien, C., et al. (2011). Harnessing neuroplasticity for clinical applications. *Brain, 134*, 1591–1609.

Curran, L. K., Newschaffer, C. J., Lee, L., Crawford, S. O., Johnston, M. V., & Zimmerman, A. W. (2007). Behaviors associated with fever in children with autism spectrum disorders. *Pediatrics, 120*(6), E1386–E1392.

Dalton, K. M., Nacewicz, B. M., Alexander, A. L., & Davidson, R. J. (2007). Gaze-fixation, brain activation, and amygdala volume in unaffected siblings of individuals with autism. *Biological Psychiatry, 61*(4), 512–520.

Dalton, K. M., Nacewicz, B. M., Johnstone, T., Schaefer, H. S., Gernsbacher, M. A., Goldsmith, H. H., & Davidson, R. J. (2005). Gaze fixation and the neural circuitry of face processing in autism. *Nature Neuroscience, 8*(4), 519–526.

Davidson, R., & McEwen, B. (2012). Social influences on neuroplasticity: Stress and interventions to promote well-being. *Nature Neuroscience, 15*(5), 689.

Dawson, G. (2008). Early behavioral intervention, brain plasticity, and the prevention of autism spectrum disorder. *Development and Psychopathology, 20*(3), 775–803.

Dawson, G. (2012). New findings hold promise for revolutionary pre-symptom screening. Autism Speaks Official Blog. Retrieved from http://blog.autismspeaks.org/.

Dawson, G., & Lewy, A. (1989). Reciprocal subcortical–cortical influences in autism: The role of attentional mechanisms (G. Dawson, Ed.). In *Autism: Nature, diagnosis, and treatment* (pp. 144–175). New York: Guilford Press.

Dawson, G., Webb, S. J., Wijsman, E., Schellenberg, G., Estes, A., Munson, J., & Faja, S. (2005). Neurocognitive and electrophysiological evidence of altered face processing in parents of children with autism: Implications for a model of abnormal development of social brain circuitry in autism. *Development and Psychopathology, 17*(3), 679–97.

Dawson, G., Jones, E. J., Merkle, K., Venema, K., Lowry, R., Faja, S., Kamara, D., Murias, M., Greenson, J., Winter, J., Smith, M., Rogers, S., & Webb, S. J. (2012). Early behavioral intervention is associated with normalized brain activity in young children with autism. *Journal of the American Academy of Child & Adolescent Psychiatry, 51*(11), 1150–1159.

DiCicco-Bloom, E., Lord, C., Zwaigenbaum, L., Courchesne, E., Dager, S., Schmitz, C., & Jan, L. (2006). The developmental neurobiology of autism spectrum disorder. *Journal of Neuroscience, 26*(26), 6897–6906.

Doidge, N. (2007). *The brain that changes itself: Stories of personal triumph from the frontiers of brain science*. New York: Viking.

Domes, G., Heinrichs, M., Michel, A., Berger, C., & Herpertz, S. C. (2007a). Oxytocin improves "mind-reading" in humans. *Biological Psychiatry, 61*(6), 731–733.

Domes, G., Heinrichs, M., Gläscher, J., Büchel, C., Braus, D. F., & Herpertz, S. C. (2007b). Oxytocin attenuates amygdala responses to emotional faces regardless of valence. *Biological Psychiatry, 62*(10), 1187–1190.

Evers, M., & Hollander, E. (2008). Excitotoxicity in autism: The role of glutamate and pathogenesis and treatment. In A. W. Zimmerman (ed.), *Autism: Current theories and evidence* (pp. 133–145). Totowa, NJ: Humana Press.

Farb, N. S., Anderson, A. K., Mayberg, H., Bean, J., McKeon, D., & Segal, Z. V. (2010). Minding one's emotions: Mindfulness training alters the neural expression of sadness. Correction to Farb et al. *Emotion, 10*(2), 215–215.

Fischbach, G. (2010, January 11). Director's column: Fever's promising puzzle. Simons Foundation Autism Research Initiative. from http://sfari.org/.

Gallese, V. (2006). Intentional attunement: A neurophysiological perspective on social cognition and its disruption in autism. *Brain Research, 1079*(1), 15–24.

Geschwind, D. H., & Levitt, P. (2007). Autism spectrum disorders: Developmental disconnection syndromes. *Current Opinion in Neurobiology, 17*(1), 103–111.

Goldapple, K. (2004). Modulation of cortical-limbic pathways in major depression: Treatment-specific effects of cognitive behavior therapy. *Archives of General Psychiatry, 61*(1), 34–41.

Gotts, S., Simmons, W., Milbury, L., Wallace, G., Cox, R., & Martin, A. (2012). Fractionation of social brain circuits in Autism Spectrum Disorders. *Brain*, 1–15.

Greenspan, S. (1992). *Infancy and early childhood: The practice of clinical assessment and intervention with emotional and developmental challenges*. Madison: International Universities Press, Inc.

Greenspan, S. I., & Shanker, S. (2004). *The first idea: How symbols, language, and intelligence evolved from our early primate ancestors to modern humans*. Cambridge, MA: Da Capo Press.

Greenspan, S. I., & Wieder, S. (1997). Developmental patterns and outcomes in infants and children with disorders in relating and communicating: A chart review of 200 cases of children with autistic spectrum diagnoses. *Journal of Developmental and Learning Disorders, 1*, 87–142.

Greenspan, S. I., & Wieder, S. (2006). *Engaging autism: Using the floortime approach to help children relate, communicate, and think.* Cambridge, MA: Da Capo Lifelong Books.

Gregory, S. G., Connelly, J. J., Towers, A. J., Johnson, J., Biscocho, D., Markunas, C. A., & Pericak-Vance, M. A. (2009). Genomic and epigenetic evidence for oxytocin receptor deficiency in autism. *BMC Medicine, 7*(1), 62.

Guastella, A. J., Einfeld, S. L., Gray, K. M., Rinehart, N. J., Tonge, B. J., Lambert, T. J., & Hickie, I. B. (2010). Intranasal oxytocin improves emotion recognition for youth with autism spectrum disorders. *Biological Psychiatry, 67*(7), 692–694.

Guastella, A. J., Mitchell, P. B., & Dadds, M. R. (2008). Oxytocin increases gaze to the eye region of human faces. *Biological Psychiatry, 63*(1), 3–5.

Hallmayer, J. S., Cleveland, A., & Torres et al. (2011). Genetic heritability and shared environmental factors among twin pairs with autism. *Archives of Gen. Psychiatry, 68*(11), 1095–1102.

Hebb, D. O. (1949). *The organization of behavior: A neuropsychological theory*. New York: John Wiley & Sons.

Helt, M., Kelley, E., Kinsbourne, M., Pandey, J., Boorstein, H., Herbert, M., & Fein, D. (2008). Can children with autism recover? If so, how? *Neuropsychology Review, 18*(4), 339–366.

Herbert, M. R. (2005a). Autism biology and the environment. *Medicine Journal of the San Francisco Medical Society, 78*(8), 13–16.

Herbert, M. R. (2005b). Large brains in autism: The challenge of pervasive abnormality. *The Neuroscientist, 11*(5), 417–440.

Herbert, M. R. (2010a). Autism: The centrality of active pathophysiology and the shift from static to chronic dynamic encephalopathy. In A. Chauhan, V. Chauhan, and T. Brown (eds.), *Autism: Oxidative stress, inflammation, and immune abnormalities* (343–387). Boca Raton, FL: Taylor & Francis.

Herbert, M. R. (2010b). Contributions of the environment and environmentally vulnerable physiology to autism spectrum disorders. *Current Opinion in Neurology, 23*(2), 103–110.

Herbert, M. R., Ziegler, D. A., Makris, N., Filipek, P. A., Kemper, T. L., Normandin, J. J., & Caviness, V. S. (2004). Localization of white matter volume increase in autism and developmental language disorder. *Annals of Neurology, 55*(4), 530–540.

Herbert, M., & Anderson, M. (2008). An expanding spectrum of autism models: From fixed developmental defects to reversible functional impairments. In A. W. Zimmerman, *Autism: Current theories and evidence* (pp. 429–463). Totowa, NJ: Humana Press.

Herbert, M. R., & Weintraub, K. (2012). *The autism revolution: Whole-body strategies for making life all it can be*. New York: Ballantine Books.

Hirstein, W., Iversen, P., & Ramachandran, V. S. (2001). Autonomic responses of autistic children to people and objects. *Proceedings of the Royal Society of London. Series B: Biological Sciences, 268*(1479), 1883–1888.

Hofer, M., & Sullivan, R. (2001). Toward a neurobiology of attachment. In C. Nelson & M. Luciana (eds.), *Handbook of developmental cognitive neuroscience* (pp. 379–392). Cambridge: M.I.T. Press.

Hollander, E., Bartz, J., Chaplin, W., Phillips, A., Sumner, J., Soorya, L., & Wasserman, S. (2007). Oxytocin increases retention of social cognition in autism. *Biological Psychiatry, 61*(4), 498–503.

Hollander, E., Novotny, S., Hanratty, M., Yaffe, R., De Caria, C., Aronowitz, B., & Mosovich, S. (2003). Oxytocin infusion reduces repetitive behaviors in adults with autistic and Asperger's disorders. *Neuropsychopharmacology, 28*, 193–198.

Insel, T. R. (1997). A neurobiological basis of social attachment. *American Journal of Psychiatry, 154*(6), 726–735.

Insel, T. R. (2010). The challenge of translation in social neuroscience: A review of oxytocin, vasopressin, and affiliative behavior. *Neuron, 65*(6), 768–779.

Jacob, S., Brune, C. W., Carter, C., Leventhal, B. L., Lord, C., & Cook Jr., E. H. (2007). Association of the oxytocin receptor gene (OXTR) in Caucasian children and adolescents with autism. *Neuroscience Letters, 417*(1), 6-9.

Kana, R., Keller, T., Cherkassky, V., Minshew, N., & Just, M. A. (2008). Atypical frontal-posterior synchronization of Theory of Mind regions in autism during mental state attribution. *Social Neuroscience, 4*(2), 135-152.

Kandel, E. (1983). From metapsychology to molecular biology: Explorations into the nature of anxiety. *American Journal of Psychiatry, 140*(10), 1277-1293.

Kandel, E. R. (1979). Psychotherapy and the single synapse. *New England Journal of Medicine, 301*(19), 1028-1037.

Keller, T. A., & Just, M. A. (2009). Altering cortical connectivity: Remediation-induced changes in the white matter of poor readers. *Neuron, 64*(5), 624-631.

Kennedy, S. H., Konarski, J. Z., Segal, Z. V., Lau, M. A., Bieling, P. J., McIntyre, R. S., & Mayberg, H. S. (2007). Differences in brain glucose metabolism between responders to CBT and venlafaxine in a 16-week randomized controlled trial. *American Journal of Psychiatry, 164*(5), 778–788.

Kinney, D., Munir, K., Crowley, D., & Miller, A. (2008b). Prenatal stress and risk for autism. *Neuroscience & Biobehavioral Reviews, 32*(8), 1519–1532.

Kinney, D., Andrea, K., Miller, M., Crowley, D. J., Huang, E., & Gerber, E. (2008a). Autism prevalence following prenatal exposure to hurricanes and tropical storms in Louisiana. *Journal of Autism and Developmental Disorders 38*(3), 481–488.

Kinsbourne, M., & Helt, M. 2011. Entrainment, mimicry, and interpersonal synchrony. In D. Fein (ed). 2011. *The neuropsychology of autism*. 1st ed. New York: Oxford University Press.

Kinsbourne, M.(1987). Cerebral-brainstem relations in infantile autism. In E. Schopler & G. B. Mesibov (eds.). *Neurobiological issues in autism*. (pp.107–125). New York: Plenum Press.

Kleinhans, N. M., Johnson, L. C., Richards, T., Mahurin, R., Greenson, J., Dawson, G., & Aylward, E. (2009). Reduced neural habituation in the amygdala and social impairments in Autism Spectrum Disorders. *American Journal of Psychiatry, 166*(4), 467–475.

Kliman, G. (2011). *Reflective network therapy in the preschool classroom* (E. Burian, Contributing Ed.). Lanham, MD: University Press of America.

Kosfeld, M., Heinrichs, M., Zak, P. J., Fischbacher, U., & Fehr, E. (2005). Oxytocin increases trust in humans. *Nature, 435*(7042), 673–676.

LeDoux, J. E. (2000). Emotion circuits in the brain. *Annual Review of Neuroscience, 23*(1), 155–184.

Lerer, E., Levi, S., Salomon, S., Darvasi, A., Yirmiya, N., & Ebstein, R. P. (2007). Association between the oxytocin receptor (OXTR) gene and autism: Relationship to Vineland Adaptive Behavior Scales and cognition. *Molecular Psychiatry, 13*(10), 980–988.

Lewis, M., Tanimura, Y., Lee, L., & Bodfish, J. (2007). Animal models of restricted repetitive behavior in autism. *Behavioural Brain Research, 176*(1), 66–74.

Lewis, Marc D. Self-organizing individual differences in brain development. *Developmental Review 25*(3–4) (2005): 252–277.

Liu, X., Kawamura, Y., Shimada, T., Otowa, T., Koishi, S., Sugiyama, T., & Sasaki, T. (2010). Association of the oxytocin receptor (OXTR) gene polymorphisms with Autism Spectrum Disorder (ASD) in the Japanese population. *Journal of Human Genetics, 55*(3), 137–141.

Loman, M., & Gunnar, M. (2010). Early experience and the development of stress reactivity and regulation in children. *Neurosci. Biobehav. Rev., 34*(6), 867–876.

Mahler, M. S. (1968). *On human symbiosis and the vicissitudes of individuation*. New York: International Universities Press.

Markram, K. (2010). Intense World Syndrome—an alternative theory of autism. PowerPoint.

Markram, H., Rinaldi, T., & Markram, K. (2007). The Intense World Syndrome—an alternative hypothesis for autism. *Front Neurosci., 1*(1), 77–96.

Markram, K., Rinaldi, T., La Mendola, D., Sandi, C. and Markram, H. (2008). Abnormal fear conditioning and amygdala processing in an animal model of autism. *Neuropsychopharmacology, 33*(4), 901–912.

Markram K., & Markram H. (2010). The Intense World Theory—a unifying theory of the neurobiology of autism. *Front. Hum. Neurosci.* 4, 224.

Mazefsky, C., Pelphrey, K., & Dahl, R. (2012). The need for a broader approach to emotion regulation research and autism. *Child Development Perspectives,* 1–6.

McEwen, B. (2006). Protective and damaging effects of stress mediators: Central role of the brain. *Dialogues Clin. Neurosci., 8*, 367–381.

McEwen, B., & Lasley, E. (2002). *The end of stress as we know it.* Washington, DC: Joseph Henry Press.

McEwen, B., & Tucker, P. (2011). Critical biological pathways for chronic psychosocial stress and research opportunities to advance the consideration of stress in chemical risk assessment. *American Journal of Public Health, 101*, S131–S139.

McEwen, B., & Wingfield, J. (2003). The concept of allostasis in biology and biomedicine. *Hormones and Behavior, 43*, 2–15.

Meaney, M., LeDoux, J., & Liebowitz, M. (2008). Neurobiology of anxiety disorders. In A. Tasman, J. Kay, & J. A. Lieberman, et al. (eds.), *Psychiatry* (pp. 317–338). Chichester, West Sussex, England: John Wiley & Sons.

Mehler, M. F., & Purpura, D. P. (2009). Autism, fever, epigenetics and the locus coeruleus. *Brain Research Reviews, 59*(2), 388–392.

Minshew, N., Williams, D., & McFadden, K. (2008). Information processing, neural connectivity, and neuronal organization. In A. W. Zimmerman (ed,), *Autism: Current theories and evidence* (pp. 381–405). Totowa, NJ: Humana Press.

Moorman, D. (2010, April 1). Workshop report: Fever and autism. Simons Foundation Autism Research Initiative. from http://sfari.org/.

Morgan, K. (2006). Is autism a stress disorder? What studies of nonautistic populations can tell us. In M. Baron, L. Lipsitt, J. Groden, & G. Groden (eds.), *Stress and coping in autism* (pp. 129–182). Oxford: Oxford University Press.

Moriceau, S., & Sullivan, R. M. (2005). Neurobiology of infant attachment. *Developmental Psychobiology, 47*(3), 230–242.

Mosconi, M., Cody-Hazlett, H., Poe, M., Gerig, G., Gimpel-Smith, R., & Piven, J. (2009). Longitudinal study of amygdala volume and joint attention in 2- to 4-year old children with autism. *Arch. Gen. Psychiatry, 66*(5), 509–516.

Mundy, P. (2003). Annotation: The neural basis of social impairments in autism: The role of the dorsal medial-frontal cortex and anterior cingulate system. *Journal of Child Psychology and Psychiatry, 44*(6), 793–809.

Nacewicz, B. M., Dalton, K. M., Johnstone, T., Long, M. T., McAuliff, E. M., Oakes, T. R., & Davidson, R. J. (2006). Amygdala volume and nonverbal social impairment in adolescent and adult males with autism. *Archives of General Psychiatry, 63*(12), 1417–1428.

Nakatani, J., Tamada, K., Hatanaka, F., Ise, S., Ohta, H., Inoue, K., & Banerjee, R. (2009). Abnormal behavior in a chromosome-engineered mouse model for human 15q11-13 duplication seen in autism. *Cell, 137*(7), 1235–1246.

Narayanan, A., White, C. A., Saklayen, S., Scaduto, M. J., Carpenter, A. L., Abduljalil, A., & Beversdorf, D. Q. (2010). Effect of propranolol on functional connectivity in Autism Spectrum Disorder—A pilot study. *Brain Imaging and Behavior, 4*(2), 189–197.

National Scientific Council on the Developing Child (2010). Early experiences can alter gene expression and affect long-term development: Working paper no. 10. Retrieved from: www.developingchild.net.

Oberman, L. M., & Ramachandran, V. S. (2007). The simulating social mind: The role of the mirror neuron system and simulation in the social and communicative deficits of autism spectrum disorders. *Psychological Bulletin, 133*(2), 310–327.

Ochsner, K., & Gross, J. (2005). The cognitive control of emotion. *Trends in Cognitive Sciences, 9*(5), 242–249.

Ochsner, K. N., Ray, R. D., Cooper, J. C., Robertson, E. R., Chopra, S., Gabrieli, J. D., & Gross, J. J. (2004). For better or for worse: Neural systems supporting the cognitive down- and up-regulation of negative emotion. *NeuroImage, 23*(2), 483–499.

Panksepp, J. (1998). *Affective neuroscience: The foundations of human and animal emotions.* New York: Oxford University Press.

Panksepp, J., Nelson, E., & Bekkedal, M. (1997). Brain systems for the mediation of social separation-distress and social-reward. *Annals of the New York Academy of Sciences, 807*(1 Integrative N), 78–100.

Pascual-Leone, A., Tarazona, F., Keenan, J., Tormos, J., Hamilton, R., & Catala, M. (1998). Transcranial magnetic stimulation and neuroplasticity. *Neuropsychologia, 37*(2), 207–217.

Pelphrey, K. A., & Carter, E. J. (2008). Charting the typical and atypical development of the social brain. *Development and Psychopathology, 20*(04), 1081–1102.
Perry, B. D. (2006). Applying principles of neurodevelopment to clinical work with maltreated and traumatized children: The neurosequential model of therapeutics. In N. B. Webb (ed.). *Working with traumatized children and youth in child welfare* (p. 27). New York: The Guilford Press.
Pessah, I., & Lein, P. (2008). Evidence for environmental susceptibility in autism: What we need to know about gene x environment interactions. In A. W. Zimmerman (ed.), *Autism: Current Theories and Evidence* (pp. 409–428). Totowa, NJ: Humana.
Popoli, M., Yan, Z., McEwen, B., & Sanacora, G. (2011). The stressed synapse: the impact of stress and glucocorticoids on glutamate transmission. *Nat. Rev. Neurosci., 13*(1), 22–37.
Porges, S. (2009). The polyvagal theory: New insights into adaptive reactions of the autonomic nervous system. *Cleveland Clinic Journal of Medicine, 76*(2), S86–S90.
Porges, S. W. (2004/2011). Neuroception: A subconscious system for detecting threat and safety. In S. W. Porges (ed.), *The polyvagal theory: Neurophysiological foundations of emotions, attachment, communication, and self-regulation* (pp. 11–19). New York: W. W. Norton.
Porges, S. W. (1993/2011). The infant's sixth sense: Awareness and regulation of bodily processes. In S. W. Porges (ed.), *The polyvagal theory: Neurophysiological foundations of emotions, attachment, communication, and self-regulation* (pp. 75–82). New York: W. W. Norton.
Porges, S. W., Doussard-Roosevelt, J. A., & Maiti, A. K. (1994/2011a). Vagal tone and the physiological regulation of emotion. In S. W. Porges (ed.), *The polyvagal theory: Neurophysiological foundations of emotions, attachment, communication, and self-regulation* (pp. 133–150). New York: W. W. Norton.
Porges, S. W. (1994/2011b). The vagus: A mediator of behavioral and physiologic features associated with autism. In S. W. Porges (Ed.) *The polyvagal theory: Neurophysiological foundations of emotions, attachment, communication, and self-regulation* (pp. 217–225). New York: W. W. Norton.
Porges, S. W. (1998/2011). Love: An emergent property of the mammalian autonomic nervous system. In S. W. Porges (Ed.) *The polyvagal theory: Neurophysiological foundations of emotions, attachment, communication, and self-regulation* (pp. 167–185). New York: W. W. Norton.
Ramachandran, V. (2011). *The tell-tale brain*. New York: W.W. Norton.
Ramachandran, V., & Oberman, L. (2006). "Broken mirrors: A theory of autism." *Scientific American 295*(5), 62–69.
Rinaldi, T., Perrodin, C., & Markram, H. (2008). Hyperconnectivity and hyperplasticity in the medial prefrontal cortex in the valproic acid animal model of autism. *Frontiers in Neural Circuits, 2*(4).
Robison, J. E. (2011). *Be different: Adventures of a free-range Aspergian with practical advice for Aspergians, misfits, families & teachers*. New York: Crown Archetype.
Rodrigues, S. M., Saslow, L. R., Garcia, N., John, O. P., & Keltner, D. (2009). Oxytocin receptor genetic variation relates to empathy and stress reactivity in humans. *Proceedings of the National Academy of Sciences,106*(50), 21437–21441.
Rogers, S., & Dawson, G. (2010). *Early Start Denver Model for young children with autism*. New York: Guilford Press, 77.
Rossman, I., & DiCicco-Bloom, E. (2008). ENGRAILED2 and cerebellar development in the pathogenesis of Autism Spectrum Disorders. In A. W. Zimmerman (ed.), *Autism: Current theories and evidence* (pp. 3–33). Totowa, NJ: Humana Press.
Sapolsky, R. (1998). *Why zebras don't get ulcers: A guide to stress, stress related diseases and coping*. New York: W. H. Freeman.
Sapolsky, R. (2005). *Biology and human behavior*. Chantilly, VA: Teaching Co..
Sapolsky, R. 2010. *Stress and your body*. Chantilly, VA: Teaching Co..
Schmahmann, J. (2010). The role of the cerebellum in cognition and emotion: Personal reflections since 1982 on the dysmetria of thought hypothesis, and its historical evolution from theory to therapy. *Neuropsychol. Rev., 20*, 236–260.

Scott-Van Zeeland, A. A., Abrahams, B. S., Alvarez-Retuerto, A. I., Sonnenblick, L. I., Rudie, J. D., Ghahremani, D., & Bookheimer, S. Y. (2010). Altered functional connectivity in frontal lobe circuits is associated with variation in the autism risk gene CNTNAP2. *Science Translational Medicine, 2*(56), 56ra80–56ra80.

Settlage, C. (1992). Psychoanalytic observations on adult development in life and in the therapeutic relationship. *Psychoanalysis and Contemporary Thought, 15*, 349–374.

Shackman, A., Maxwell, J., Mcmenamin, B., Greischar, L., & Davidson, R. (2011). Stress potentiates early and attenuates late stages of visual processing. *The Journal of Neuroscience, 31* (3), 1156–1161.

Sherkow, S. (2005). Psychoanalytic approaches to working with children with autism spectrum disorder: Case report by Dr. Susan Sherkow of 2-1/2-year-old boy in dyadic psychoanalytic treatment. Paper presented at American Psychoanalytic Association Meeting Winter 2005, Waldorf-Astoria Hotel, New York.

Sherkow, S. P. (2007). Personal communication.

Sherkow, S. P. (2011). The dyadic psychoanalytic treatment of a toddler with autism spectrum disorder. *Psychoanalytic Inquiry, 31*, 252–275.

Siegel, D. J. (2007). *The mindful brain: Reflection and attunement in the cultivation of well-being*. New York: W.W. Norton.

Singletary, W. M. (2006, February 21). Forget the stage fright, just play the music: The psychoanalytic treatment of children with ASD. Lecture presented at Margaret S. Mahler Child Psychotherapy Lecture at Psychoanalytic Center of Philadelphia, Philadelphia, Pennsylvania.

Singletary, W. M. (2009, January 14). Introduction: Psychoanalytic approaches to autistic spectrum disorder: Extending the dialogue between psychoanalysis and neurobiology. Lecture presented at discussion group: Winter meeting of the American Psychoanalytic Association, New York, New York.

Spencer, M., Holt, R., Chura, L., et al. (2011). A novel functional brain imaging endophenotype autism: The neural response to facial expression of emotion. *Translational Psychiatry, 1*(E19).

Spitz, R. (1945). Hospitalism—An inquiry into the genesis of psychiatric conditions in early childhood. *Psychoanal. St. Child, 1*, 53–74.

Spitz, R. (1955). The primal cavity—A contribution to the genesis of perception and its role for psychoanalytic theory. *The Psychoanalytic Study of the Child, 10*, 215–240.

Sullivan, R. (2003). Developing a sense of safety: The neurobiology of neonatal attachment. *Annals of the New York Academy of Sciences, 1008*, 122–131.

Szalavitz, M., & Perry, B. D. (2010). *Born for love: Why empathy is essential—and endangered*. New York: William Morrow.

Szatmari, P. (2011). Is autism, at least in part, a disorder of fetal programming? *Archives of Gen. Psychiatry, 68*(11), 1091–1092.

Tansey, K. E., Brookes, K. J., Hill, M. J., Cochrane, L. E., Gill, M., Skuse, D., & Gallagher, L. (2010). Oxytocin receptor (OXTR) does not play a major role in the aetiology of autism: Genetic and molecular studies. *Neuroscience Letters, 474*(3), 163–167.

Taub, E., Ramey, S. L., DeLuca, S., & Echols, K. (2004). Efficacy of constraint-induced movement therapy for children with cerebral palsy with asymmetric motor impairment. *Pediatrics, 113*(2), 305–312.

Taub, E. (2008). "Brain Science Podcast." Interview by Ginger Campbell. Audio blog post. Brain science podcast with Ginger Campbell. Episode #28. Web. 11 Jan. 2008.

Teicher, M. H., Polcari, A., Andersen, S. L., Anderson, C. M., & Navalta, C. (2003). Neurobiological effects of childhood stress and trauma. In S. W. Coates, J. L. Rosenthal, & D. S. Schechter (eds.), *September 11: Trauma and human bonds* (pp. 211–238). The Analytic Press/Taylor & Francis Group.

Thompson, B., & Levitt, P. (2010). Now you see it, now you don't—Closing in on allostasis and developmental basis of psychiatric disorders. *Neuron, 65*, 437.

Tottenham, N., & Sheridan, M. (2010). A review of adversity, the amygdala and the hippocampus: A consideration of developmental timing. *Frontiers in Human Neuroscience, 3*.

Tronick, E., & Beeghley, M. (2011). Infants' meaning-making and the development of mental health problems. *American Psychologist, 66*(2), 107–119.
Tustin, F. (1990). *The protective shell in children and adults*. London: Karnac Books.
Valentino, R., & Van Bockstaele, E. (2008). Convergent regulation of locus coeruleus activity as an adaptive response to stress. *European Journal of Pharmacology, 583*, 194–203.
Van Bockstaele, E., Bajic, D., Proudfit, H., & Valentino, R. (2001). Topographic architecture of stress-related pathways targeting the noradrenergic locus coeruleus. *Physiol. Behav., 73*(3), 273–83.
Van Der Kolk, B. (2013). Foreward. In S. Porges (ed.) (2011). *The polyvagal theory: Neurophysiological foundations of emotions, attachment, communication, and self-regulation* (pp. xi–xvii). 1st ed. New York: W. W. Norton & Company.
Vrtička, P., Andersson, F., Grandjean, D., Sander, D., & Vuilleumier, P. (2008). Individual attachment style modulates human amygdala and striatum activation during social appraisal (P. Zak, Ed.). *PLoS ONE, 3*(8), E2868.
Wager, T., Davidson, M., Hughes, B., Lindquist, M., & Ochsner, K. (2008). Prefrontal-subcortical pathways mediating successful emotional regulation. *Neuron, 59*, 1037–1050.
Waterhouse, L. (2008). Autism overflows: Increasing prevalence and proliferating theories. *Neuropsychol. Rev., 18*, 273–286.
Waterhouse, L. (2013). *Rethinking autism*. London: Academic Press.
Wieder, S., Greenspan, S., & Kalmanson, B. (2008). Autism assessment and intervention: The developmental individual-difference, relationship-based DIR® / Floortime™ Model. *Zero to Three, 28*(4), 31–37.
Williams, D. (2008). What neuroscience has taught us about autism. *Zero to Three, 28*(4), 11–17.
Wismer Fries, A., Ziegler, T., Kurian, J., Jacoris, S., & Pollack, S. (2005). Early experience in humans is associated with changes in neuropeptides critical for regulating social behavior. *PNAS, 102*(47), 17237–17240.
Wolff, J., Gu, H., Gerig, G., et al. For the IBIS Network. (2012). Differences in white matter fiber tract development present from 6 to 24 months in infants with autism. *American Journal of Psychiatry, 169*, 589–600.
Wu, S., Jia, M., Ruan, Y., Liu, J., Guo, Y., Shuang, M., & Zhang, D. (2005). Positive association of the oxytocin receptor gene (OXTR) with autism in the Chinese Han population. *Biological Psychiatry, 58*(1), 74–77.
Zaki, J., & Ochsner, K. (2009). The need for a cognitive neuroscience of naturalistic social cognition. *Ann. N.Y. Acad. Sci., 1167*, 16–30.
Zaki, J., & Ochsner, K. (2011). Reintegrating the study of accuracy into social cognition research. *Psychological Inquiry, 22*(3), 159–182.
Zaki, J., & Ochsner, K. (2012). The cognitive neuroscience of sharing and understanding others' emotions. In J. Decety (ed.), *Empathy: From bench to bedside* (pp. 207–226). Cambridge: MIT Press.
Zaki, J., Hennigan, K., Weber, J., & Ochsner, K. (2010). Social cognitive conflict resolution: Contributions of domain-general and domain-specific neural systems. *The Journal of Neuroscience, 30*(25), 8481–8488.
Zaki, J., Weber, J., Bolger, N., & Ochsner, K. (2009). The neural bases of empathic accuracy. *Proceedings of the National Acadmey of Sciences, 106*(20), 11382–11387.
Zimmerman, A. W. (2008). *Autism: Current theories and evidence.* Totowa, NJ: Humana Press.

DISCUSSION

Ablon, S. L., Harrison, A. M., & Valenstein, A. F. (1986). Gifford: Special solutions to phallic-aggressive conflict in male twins. *Psychoanal. St. Child., 41*, 239–257.
Baron-Cohen, S. (1995). *Mindblindness: An essay on autism and theory of mind.* Cambridge, MA: MIT Press.

Chused, J. (1988). The transference neurosis in child analysis. *Psychoanal. St. Child., 43*, 51–81.

Dawson, G., Rogers, S., Munson, J., Smith, M., Winter, J., Donaldson, A., Greenson, J., & Varley, J. (2010). Randomized controlled trial of an intervention for toddlers with autism: The Early Start Denver Model. *Pediatrics, 125*, 1:e17–e23.

Fonagy, P., Gergely, G., Jurist, E., & Target, M. (2002). *Affect regulation, mentalization, and the development of the self.* London, Karnac Books.

Greenspan S., & Wieder, S. (2011). Relationship-based early intervention approach to autistic spectrum disorders: The DIR model. In D. G. Amaral, G. Dawson, & D. H. Geschwind (eds.), *Autism Spectrum Disorders* (pp. 1068–1080). New York: Oxford University Press.

Harrison, A. M. (forthcoming). The sandwich model of therapeutic action. *Int. J. Psychoanal.*

Harrison, A. M., & Tronick, E. (2007). Now we have a playground: Emerging new ideas of therapeutic action. *J. Amer. Psychoanal. Assoc.*, *55*(3), 853–874.

Hesse, E., & Main, M. (2000). Disorganized attachment, child and adult attachment: Collapse in behavioral and attentional strategies. *J. Amer. Psychoanal. Assoc., 48*(4), 1097–1127.

Kandel, E. (1983). From metapsychology to molecular biology: Explorations into the nature of anxiety. *Amer. J. Psychiat., 140*(10), 1277–1293.

Lieberman, A., Padron, E., Van Horn, P., & Harris, W. (2005). Angels in the nursery: The intergenerational transmission of benevolent parental influences. *J. Infant Mental Health, 26(*6), 504–520.

Modell, A. H. (1997). The synergy of memory, affects, and metaphor. *J. Anal. Psychol. 42*, 105–117.

Perry, B., & Hambrick, E. (2008). The neurosequential model of therapeutics. http://childtrauma.org/images/stories/Articles/nmt_article_08.pdf /3: 37–43.

Reddy, V. (2008). *How infants know minds*. Cambridge: Harvard University Press, 43–65.

Smolen, A. *Mothering without a home*. In Press.

Stern, D. (1985). *The interpersonal world of the infant*. New York: Basic Books, 138–161.

Trevarthen, C. (2005). Action and emotion in development of cultural intelligence: Why infants have feelings like ours. In J. Nadel & D. Muir (eds.), *Emotional development*. New York: Oxford University Press, 61–91.

Index

About the Authors

Susan P. Sherkow, MD, is a training and supervising analyst at the Berkshire Psychoanalytic Institute and Society and an Instructor in the Adult Division and Supervising Analyst in the Child Division of the New York Psychoanalytic Institute and Society. She is also an assistant clinical professor at the Mt. Sinai and Albert Einstein Colleges of Medicine and has published and presented widely on the topics of autism spectrum disorder, child development, play, infantile masturbation, and infantile eating disorders. More information about her work and private practice can be found at sherkowcenter.org.

Alexandra M. Harrison, MD, is a training and supervising analyst at the Boston Psychoanalytic Society and Institute, assistant clinical professor of psychiatry, Harvard Medical School at Cambridge Health Alliance, and on the Core Faculty of the Infant-Parent Mental Health Program at University of Massachusetts Boston. Dr. Harrison has published and presented on the treatment of autism spectrum disorders and children with uneven development, therapeutic action in psychoanalysis and psychotherapy, and supporting the caregiving relationship. She is the author of the blog www.supportingchildcaregivers.com.

William M. Singletary, MD, is a child and adult psychiatrist and psychoanalyst on the faculty of the Psychoanalytic Center of Philadelphia and President of the Board of the Margaret S. Mahler Psychiatric Research Foundation. In private practice near Philadelphia, Dr. Singletary has worked in intensive psychotherapy with children with autistic spectrum disorder for approximately 25 years.

www.ingramcontent.com/pod-product-compliance
Ingram Content Group UK Ltd.
Pitfield, Milton Keynes, MK11 3LW, UK
UKHW012038150926
475560UK00001B/77

9 780765 708625